Secrets of Successful Pranayama

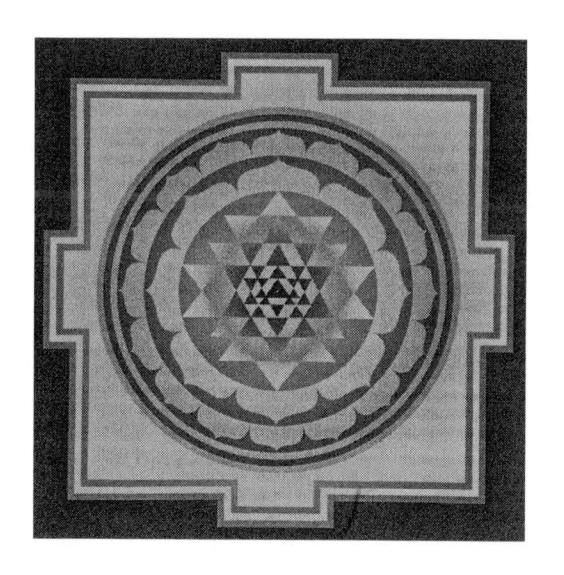

A Practical, Step-by-Step Guidebook to the Life-Transforming Practice of Yogic Breathing

VOLUME I: BASIC PRACTICES

T. Abrehamson

Copyright © 2013 T. Abrehamson
All rights reserved.
ISBN: 9780615635255
ISBN 13: 0615635253

atha

WISDOM

without power and compassion
wisdom is wasted

POWER

without wisdom and compassion
power is wasted

COMPASSION

without wisdom and power
compassion is wasted

A Few Nice Words

Tom is a masterful teacher. Before studying with him, I thought little of breathing, except for when I had a cold or was on a long run. Pranayama has become a touchstone in my daily life, bringing clarity and a sense of the now.

>Sheri Sheppard
>Professor, Mechanical Engineering
>Stanford University
>Chair, Stanford Faculty Senate, 2006-2007

Table of Contents

SECTION I

What is Pranayama?................................ 1
Why Should <u>You</u> Practice Pranayama?............... 3
How to Use This Book............................. 7
Some Useful Definitions.......................... 17

SECTION II

How to Get the Most Out of Your Practice........... 23
(1) Practice Daily 25
(2) Practice in the Early Morning 27
(3) Clean Your Systems......................... 33
(4) Calm Your Belly 41
(5) Wear Helpful Clothing...................... 45
(6) Practice for a Set Time Period............. 49

How to Settle In.................................. 55
(7) How to Use External Posture 57
(8) How to Get Quiet........................... 63
(9) How to Get Help 73

SECTION III

The Basic Pranayama.............................. 77
(10) Energy 101................................ 79
(11) Pranayama 101 93

(12) Kapalabhati 101
(13) Nadi Shodana. 121
(14) Agni Sara. 151
(15) Asvini Mudra. 159
(16) Ujjayi 165

How to Finish. 173
(17) Sitting: Meditation Variations 175
(18) Lying Down: "Perfection". 187

SECTION IV

Health Benefits of Yoga & Pranayama 199
    Freedom from Sickness 199
    Life-Extension & Anti-Aging. 200
    Pranayama & Calm in Your Life 201
    Weight Control from Pranayama? 202
    Respiratory Capacity 203

Pranayama, Asana & Energy 205

Other Pranayama Books? 211

THE BIG PICTURE. 213

Your Work 217

Our Aim 219

What is "Pranayama?"

"Pranayama" is Yogic Breathing, a great variety of practices. It is just one part of various "Yoga" systems, some of which are thousands of years old.

"Prana" refers to a Subtle Vital Energy, an Energy not yet often recognized by Western science but which some Eastern thinking believes to be pervasive. "Life-Force" might be one acceptable interpretation. "Yama" can refer to regulation, restraint; its Sanskrit root word refers to reins or bridles. We might therefore say that with Pranayama we harness Universal Energy by regulating our breath.

This is of course an extremely important assertion. You can test its validity. This Guidebook is designed to teach you the basics of Pranayama.

In Sanskrit, if an "a" is put in the front of the word "yama" the resultant word can be said to refer to "stretching" or "expansion," (the opposite of "restraint.") In this context, "Pranayama" may, in one sense, allude to the expansion of Energy, or the stretching of Energy, as in up from the bottom of the torso to the top of the body. This is sometimes referred to, in some of its aspects, as "Kundalini rising."

The Sanskrit base of the word "Kundalini" can mean "coiled." A pool of Vital Energy is thus considered, in some Yogic thought, as latent, like a coiled snake, in the area of the tailbone. And the word "Kundalini" is therefore often used in the context of a snake uncoiling, rising up and expanding (like a cobra), in order to portray the blossoming of that Energy - and Kundalini is depicted pictographically as a cobra.

The Pranayama set forth in <u>Secrets of Successful Pranayama</u>, therefore, in working to harness/utilize Energy, strive, in part, to make Energy rise up/expand from the lower abdomen in order to effectuate its full use.

The above discussion should help you to understand that to think of Pranayama as merely "Yogic breathing exercises" is an oversimplification that omits the most important aspects of the practice.

Breath is a Key that Unlocks Us.

Why Should <u>You</u> Practice Pranayama?

On one level: Pranayama can make you Feel Great: utterly calm and quiet, light yet grounded, and confident and empowered. Pranayama is also a wonderful lead-in to Meditation and adds to its success and depth. Further, it opens the body for improved progress in Yoga poses, ("Asana").

This is all nice, yes. But, relatively, minor.

On a higher level: Pranayama is Life-Transforming. It links you up with the Universe. You trend in the right direction. Things start to knit together, to slot into place more easily. Your day and your life can flow more smoothly, with economy of effort. Intuitions flow like rain. Your mistakes can become less bothersome and more amusing. You can fix rather than fume. Nagging irritants can spontaneously heal/disappear. You can accept correct decisions. You can become more even-keeled. You can ground. You can stay more on-track. You can be in fact empowered. You can be open to becoming more purpose-full, more use-full.

Reaping these rewards are what I mean by Successful Pranayama. And yes, at first all this can sound incredibly mystical and otherworldly. But my personal experiences are in harmony with those of others, over the centuries.

With Persistent Practice
Your life will change for the better.
Spontaneously, effortlessly and permanently.
You are becoming whole. Becoming what you should be.
You are forging an instrument of Will.

The Big Question

Why is "just" working with our breath so hugely spiritual?
Because it Enables us. To Connect. To Yoke Up.
How does it do that?
It strips away intervening blockages.
It Purifies us.
It allows Connection and Flow.

This is the most important section in this book.

Legal Disclaimer
Important! Read This!

The materials and content contained in this book are not intended to be, nor are they, a substitute for professional medical health care, advice, diagnosis or treatment. They are not meant to replace the advice of health care professionals. The information contained herein reflects the lay opinion of the writer. It is in no way to be considered as professional medical advice.

Never disregard professional medical advice, or rely on the information contained in this book in place of seeking professional medical advice regarding your own health needs. Any and all medical questions you have should be presented to your own licensed health care provider.

Working with the breath can entail physical and/or mental risk.

It is thus your responsibility to ascertain – by reviewing your practice intentions carefully with your licensed health care provider prior to beginning the practices described herein – that there is no medical reason to prevent you from undertaking any specific practice.

Pregnant Women!

It is YOUR responsibility to protect yourself and your fetus.

Do not undertake the practices described in this book without first discussing your intentions with a licensed health care provider, and getting their professional assent to your proposed practice.

How to Use this Book

Overview of the Guidebook

This Guidebook consists of four helpful sections:
This FIRST section introduces you to Pranayama and to the Guidebook.
The SECOND tells you how to set up your own practice.
The THIRD tells you what to do during your practice.
The FOURTH tells you some benefits to expect.

The Guidebook describes many Pranayama. Please treat them as a <u>Menu</u>, not as a <u>Prescription</u>. You may pick and choose among them for any particular practice.

Your Study Manual

This is not a quick-fix handbook. This is not an executive summary with bullet points. This is not "Yoga-Lite." This is a study manual and a reference book. It is not easily digested.

Okay. Understood. But how on earth am I supposed to remember all these instructions while I'm concentrating on my <u>breathing</u>?

Good Question! You can't. At first.

A tremendous amount of information, that came to me incrementally, over years and years and years, is being thrown at you all at once. It needs assimilation. So bring it on board, but do so in bits and pieces. Work at it. Don't expect quick perfection. Don't expect to be able to jump right into a fully developed personal practice.

This Guidebook is designed to give you a whole galaxy of options to choose from. There is enough here for you to chew on productively for years and years. Yoga can be a long, arduous path.

A Living Teacher or a Guidebook?

<u>Secrets of Successful Pranayama</u> grew out of notes I made for teaching Pranayama in my Yoga classes. It then became a handout for my Pranayama Workshops, intended as a follow-up for students to use as they continued to practice on their own. And it then blossomed into its current form: a Guidebook designed to allow you yourself to develop your own practice, at home, without the necessity of a living instructor.

There are a myriad of cautions about progressing into Pranayama without being instructed in it by a living teacher. I agree, in large part. However, more important, to my mind, is the question: Why should the wonderful benefits of Pranayama be available only to those fortunate enough to live close enough to an experienced teacher?

The aim of this work is to make Pranayama accessible to anyone, anywhere.

Give someone a Yoga Class, feed their Day.
Give someone a Yoga Guidebook, feed their Life.

<u>Secrets of Successful Pranayama</u> is intended not only for someone who has already been introduced to Pranayama, but also for someone who perhaps has little or no knowledge of Yoga but who wishes to learn about Yogic Breathing. If you are that person this is the book for you. <u>Everything you need to know to practice beginning Pranayama is set out here</u>. (And in coming years you will find guidance for Intermediate and Advanced practices in Volumes II and III.)

That said, I am firmly convinced, from experience with the students in my classes, workshops and private lessons, that instruction from a living instructor is the very best way to insure that you are on the right track. I have tried to make this Guidebook as crystal clear as possible, but my students continue to find flaws in my expositions and try to tell me, sometimes vociferously, not to go off on misguided tangents.

Get the Basics Down First

This Guidebook is designed not only to map out the main thoroughfares of a Pranayama practice for you, but also to help you delve into intriguing little alleyways and footpaths that can lead you to important discoveries.

So. Don't get lost in the clutter. Since what is being offered to you here can seem tremendously complex, the key is for you to build a solid foundation, over time, before you go deeper into the nuances. Stay simple at first.

When the basics of a particular Pranayama become second nature to you, you can build on those basics, adding more things to try to be aware of as you practice. In other words, don't overload yourself at the start by trying to remember everything. Then, once you are established in a practice, look for little things that help more.

Stick With It: 3 Weeks / 8 Weeks

A Daily Practice for Three Weeks, hopefully at the same time of the day each day, should be enough to establish Pranayama as a habit. And Eight Weeks of daily or nearly-daily practice should convince you of Pranayama's power. Hint: see how your daily life flows. Hint: see if you are becoming more conscious about how to improve your relationships with other people, and are actually attempting to do so, with some success.

Note, however, that Pranayama is not about instant gratification. And, also, that any phenomena that you might experience – even immediately – during your practice are quite nice, but that Pranayama is about the long-term building up of, and continuance of, a Purification.

To put it another way: Pranayama is not like a pill you pop for an instant fix. It is like a cream that you rub into your skin each day for long-term self-betterment.

You may be looking for your better self. Pranayama can take you there. Be patient with it. You should find yourself, over the long haul, in a virtuous spiral, in which your activities, (and perhaps even your movements), become more and more purposeful and not extraneous.

These Pranayama are Just My Recommendations

The Pranayama set forth here have been very effective for me. But they are just one person's experience, one person's versions. Proven methods, which have worked for me and for my students, and which are offered to you for your consideration.

There are, however, many other different, and valid, Pranayama methodologies. Please stray. I do, all the time. I am constantly testing and experimenting, trying out things from newly-discovered sources, and trying especially to find short Pranayama sequences which will work within the limited-time-setting of a predominantly Asana-oriented Yoga class.

Do a Varied Practice

I also suggest that you might want to vary your practice, at least somewhat, from day to day. If you do not do so it may become mechanical. You may go though the motions, but without the necessary intensity, the complete involvement every single step: every single Inhale, Retention and Exhale. Guard against sterile repetition. Think instead: "OK, today I feel like doing thus and such."

I believe it is likely that every possible breathing permutation and combination has been discovered over the centuries, and, often, codified, and thus, often, ossified. Don't fall into that trap.

Also, there is absolutely no necessity to do a large number of different Pranayama in a session. You can pick one, two, three, or more, and very beneficially spend quality time with them.

> I do however suggest that Nadi Shodana should be a part of each of your practices, (unless you have more than one session that day), no matter how advanced you become.

So. As mentioned at the beginning of this chapter, treat this Guidebook as a Menu, not a Prescription. Think of it as a buffet, a smorgasbord. Pick and choose. Experiment. Dabble. Mix and match. Find what works for you. Use my input as yeast to allow your own sequences to rise up from within you. See where you are led. Take what you are given. Receive your own Galaxies.

Meditate at Any Point

Always keep in mind that you may stop doing active Pranayama after any breath during your session, and just sit and Meditate. Sometimes it will feel absolutely <u>right</u> to cut things shorter than you had planned, and do so. ("Wow! I'm there! I'm done.") Follow where you are led.

Pranayama can be said to be designed in part to lead into and enhance Meditation. And although this Guidebook is dedicated to explaining Pranayama's procedures and benefits, it needs to be stated up front that Meditation can be an even more potent spiritual practice.

Just as Pranayama takes you deeper into spiritual growth than Asana, Meditation can take you deeper than Pranayama. And so, with that in mind, if you only have time to do only one of these three things, I suggest that you should Meditate. I do not delve here into the deeper aspects of Meditation, either as taught in the Yogic traditions or otherwise. There is plenty about it out there for you.

Glean

I write terse. This Guidebook is dense, tight-packed. Just because I say a thing with a few words, and do not revisit it, does not mean it is not of importance.

Attentiveness & Subtleties

On a related note, much of what is described here, or is asked of you, is very subtle – movements, actions, feelings – things that are going on inside of you, or things that you do in order to affect what is going on. You can develop over time, through attentiveness, the ability to pick up on these subtleties.

In one sense it's like when, instead of just hearing the words that someone is saying to you, you fully understand their complete message by being attentive not only to their words, but also to their tone of voice, their facial expression, their body language and other circumstances. With time, therefore, and diligent attentiveness during your practices, the messages of this book will come more alive to you.

Please be aware that I often struggle – as have others over the centuries – to find words to adequately express what is going on inside. Hopefully you will be able to develop the ability to pick out from my inadequacies some things with concrete relevance to what is happening to you in your own, very personal practice.

Question Everything!

Years of experimentation, trial and error and checking and rechecking of efficacy, have gone into this offering. But I cannot possibly be right 100% of the time. No one can. Please mentally preface every single thing I assert with a "<u>One Person's</u> current, limited <u>Opinion</u> is…" and also with a "Try this and see…"

Further, my own practice is constantly evolving. Tomorrow morning I may stumble upon something that elaborates on what I have already experienced… or supersedes it. This Guidebook is necessarily a snapshot-in-time of a Living, Growing Practice. Yoga is Exploration Without End.

> "There is no end to the refinement of practice and growth of understanding. Yoga has no limit or finality."
> Yoga Teacher David Swenson
> <u>Ashtanga Yoga, The Practice Manual</u> p 233

So. If your experience differs from mine, fine. Try, but verify. Test validity through your own experience. Keep practicing healthy disrespect/protective skepticism. There is no substitute for your own rock-solid Experienced Truth.

Don't Get Discouraged

Much of what I have experienced and am passing on to you may seem strange, weird, esoteric, or even utter nonsense. Especially so to someone who has not practiced Pranayama (or Asana or Meditation) in some depth and over a period of time.

If, for example, many years ago, before I had become drawn more actively into Pranayama, someone had tried to teach me the things in this book, I would have thought them – to be charitable – a bit off-kilter. And I realize that that particular reception can, fairly enough, await me here; but I am not about to ignore the clear and definitive testimony of my senses, nor the undeniable, ongoing enhancements to my own life.

So. It may be easy to get somewhat discouraged, or to slide deeper into skepticism, when things do not happen – or when you cannot <u>feel</u> them happening – anywhere near the way I am reporting to you. I will have to ask you to take it on trust that I am truthfully reporting my own experiences. And that the experiences being described are, again, not just mine but those of my students. And that, over the months and years, as you develop more inward sensitivity, you should in fact experience what we have.

<u>I am not offering you anything that I have not personally experienced.</u>

Don't Let <u>Me</u> Get in the Way

I tend to try to overly quantify and control. Notice the exact precision, (as opposed to inexact precision), herein and ask yourself whether it is a necessity or a manifestation of my personality type. (A picture is worth a thousand words: you are dealing with someone who has been known, when dieting, to on occasion measure the calories of his meals down to the individual blueberry.)

I think it is also wise to beware of my related tendency to refine things down. If something works for me I tend to refine it, and then to refine it again, in order to make things "Even More Better." But perhaps, sometimes – as you can see from the phraseology in the previous sentence – it's "Not."

And too, I tend to go into "exquisite detail" about things I judge to be helpful. But there is a fine line between "exquisite" and "excruciating." So – just go as deeply as you yourself would like to, at least initially. <u>Look for the Essence</u>. Look for the guiding principles. Don't think of this book as telling you exactly what you must do, but as showing you – with some "exquisite details" – what one person currently finds optimal.

All that said, I think my personality type may be of use to you in this situation. A personality type such as this is one you might like to have as a guide into uncharted territory – there is less propensity to exaggerate. I am not inclined to romanticize vague intuitions.

You might therefore appreciate that the person reporting things back to you has a penchant for exactitude and measured words, and a horror of inaccuracy. (As, for example, you might like the pilot of a plane in which you are riding to be very, very precise.)

There is a tremendous amount of gobbledygook out there, as well as theoretical exposition and unwarranted extrapolation. The Teacher standing at your shoulder should be able to answer with clarity your two questions:

What are we doing?
and
Why are we doing it?

I am NOT a Guru

I am in no sense a <u>guru</u>, or enlightened, or in any way entitled to "pontificate." I am a just a <u>guy</u> – a guy as full of faults as all of us, with a life chock-full of ups and downs – but whose path has led him into some knowledge of Yogic-based techniques, and who, as he is certain that these techniques have had a benevolent effect on his life, wishes therefore to share them with his fellow travelers.

Nor even, in the classic sense, might I be able to be considered a "Yogi," as I have not bought into all the perhaps hazily-defined precepts and practices of whatever that is.

Yoga and Pranayama are just tools. What I care about is what they do for my Relationship and relationships.

Many who espouse Yoga would have us delete the "relationships" part of the above sentence. I prefer to suffer.

A Scouting Report

Think of me, then – and of other "instructors" – as scouts who have found one way up the mountain and have reported back to you. But there are many ways up. I like to think of myself as a "Pranayama Explorer" and am constantly experimenting and making new discoveries.

Over the centuries many, many "mystical explorers" have trekked up this mountain and have discovered wonders, and have said to themselves "This is great! I've got to tell people about it!" And they have. Resulting – because of personal bias, cultural bias, the nature of what each individual discovered, and the apparently natural human tendency towards both personal and spiritual authoritarianism – in a vast array of guidances and descriptions and suggestions and – unfortunately – certainties.

I cannot say that anyone's personal opinions/truths are wrong for them. What I can say is that "My take differs…" And further, I have to admit that my take may even differ from itself, tomorrow. Part of the joy of life is that things can change unexpectedly, on a dime, and maybe for the better.

In this Guidebook I have mentioned other Yoga Teachers whose opinions I think are worthy of respect. I consider them knowledgeable; but that is not to say that you should consider them authoritative. There is only one true authority, and that is your body, your self.

So, in sum, I suggest you be wary of any "experts" who say "You <u>Must</u> Do <u>This</u>!" Don't fall into the abyss of needing to be <u>told</u> what is <u>right</u>. Find it for yourself, as it is on the day.

> "He points to the map and then makes sure that we go on our own journey and don't just keep looking at his finger."
>
> Yoga Teacher Cyndi Lee, (of Yoga Teacher Richard Rosen)

Some Useful Definitions

Over the centuries, in Yoga, different terms have been used to describe similar things. For example, one Teacher will put their own spin on an Asana or Pranayama, naming it something different from another Teacher. Adding to the confusion, words in Sanskrit – the ancient language in which some of the practices here were first described – lend themselves to multiple meanings.

Even further, pedantically correct pronunciations of the Sanskrit terms have morphed into modern versions that have become almost universally accepted. The definitions and pronunciations in <u>Secrets of Successful Pranayama</u> will go with the common usages, simply because they are what you yourself will most likely hear elsewhere.

Just two brief examples. You will hardly, if ever, hear:
1. "Sanskrit" pronounced correctly as "Sun-skrit."
2. "Chak-ra" pronounced correctly as "Chuk-ra."

Don't skip this section. It is necessary background. And besides that, it's interesting.

Yoga

A complex of ethical, behavioral and meditative/spiritual practices. There have been many variations throughout many centuries. Originally developed in the area of the Indian subcontinent, and now able to be thought of as distinct from but informed by Hinduism, aspects of Yoga resonate, as would be expected, through spiritual systems in other Asian cultures.

Hatha Yoga

The "physical poses" part of Yoga. And, if you think of Hatha Yoga (hah-thah yoh-gah) as a pie, then all the slices of the pie are the various schools of thought about how to do the poses. A "Hatha Yoga" class doesn't really tell you much about what to expect. Nor, other than a general shared emphasis, might other appellations, because there is so much individual difference between instructors and their methods and interpretations.

Thus, in my opinion, your <u>instructor</u> is usually more important than the <u>type</u> of Yoga you choose, because, luckily, Hatha Yoga is itself so powerful as a modality that almost any variation will bring about results. As Yoga Teacher Pattabhi Jois said so well: it is 99 per cent practice and 1 per cent theory. In other words, just practice regularly, no matter what variation(s) you choose.

Sidetrack: "Classical Yoga" & "Hatha Yoga"

You will often hear the "physical poses" aspect of Yoga being hyped as being 5,000 years old. This is at best misguided, and to my knowledge is based solely on seals from the ancient Indus Valley showing figures <u>sitting</u> in "Yogic-type" positions.

The "classic" Yoga of the Yoga Sutras of Patanjali – which includes Pranayama as one of the "eight limbs" ("asht-anga") of Yoga – dates from the second century Common Era (per Georg Feuerstein, our preeminent contemporary Yogic historian).

This "classic" or "Ashtanga" Yoga was primarily aimed at sitting –- it did not in my opinion involve doing all the various physical poses we now know and love or hate. Some of these came later, with "Hatha Yoga," a school of thought which was sympathetic to using our bodies

SOME USEFUL DEFINITIONS

for Yogic purposes. "Hatha Yoga," (in this sense), dates from much later – perhaps around 1400-1600.

Even more: the 2010 dissection of historical evidence by Yoga Scholar Mark Singleton – in his fascinating tome "Yoga Body – the Origins of Modern Posture Practice" – makes a plausible case that our present-day, internationalized "Hatha Yoga" poses practice is in fact a very recent construct indeed.

So. Should it <u>matter</u> to you when and where it came from?

Asana

(Ah-sah-nah). The singular and plural for "Yoga Pose." It is most often combined with a word that tells you what the pose is about. For example, a Yoga Teacher might say: "Let's take Trikonasana" rather than "Let's do triangle pose."

Or might say – (the one I like most) – "Find Trikonasana." If, however, "Try to Find Trikonasana" was not so unwieldy, it would be Number One for me.

Note that, like "Asana," "Pranayama" (Prah-nah-yah-mah) is also both the singular and the plural, describing a specific breathing technique, or more than one, or indeed referring to the whole system of "Yogic Breathing."

Savasana

(Shah-vah-sah-nah). The "lying-down-on-our-backs" relaxation pose usually done at the end of a Yoga class. It means "corpse pose." Some teachers don't like the connotation, and prefer to call it "relaxation pose" or some other name. However, in a real (pre-rigor-mortis) corpse all your strings have been cut; there is total limpness; and <u>this</u> is exactly what you wish to achieve.

Nadis

(Nah-dees). "Tubes" or "Pipes" in Sanskrit. Some ancients are said to have discovered that there are 72,000 (or some such) Subtle Energy Channels inside our bodies. How did they know?

In any event, one goal of Yoga is to purify the Nadis and to properly utilize the flow of Subtle Vital Energy ("Prana") through them.

Note: from here on Subtle Vital Energy "Prana" or "Ki" or "Chi" will simply be called Energy

There is some semblance of correspondence of meaning, and some sort of structural interface, between the "Nadis" of India and the "Meridians" used in Chinese acupuncture, which likewise chart the flows of Energy. Although the most well-known Meridians number only a handful, there are a myriad of "sub-Meridians," if you will, with the whole system encompassing – as the Nadis are said to do – the entire body.

Thus practitioners in both of these vast civilizations may be said to have come to perhaps essentially the same viewpoint.

Bandha

(Bahn-duh). A Bandha is a "Lock" which you apply, at different places, (in my interpretation inside your body). Locks are used, on one level, to seal Energy, so it is forced to the desired places during your practice, rather than dissipate or go into the wrong places.

There are three "major" Locks:

Mula Bandha

(Mool-uh Bahn-duh). The Root Lock. Mula refers to "root." Mula Bandha is perhaps the most important Lock in Yoga. It involves an Energetic lift in the area of the pelvic floor. Not for pregnant women.

SOME USEFUL DEFINITIONS

Uddiyana Bandha

(Oo-di-ahnah Bahn-duh). The Belly Lock. In the interpretation that I like you take the mid-section of your torso in and up. Uddiyana refers to "flying upward." This in essence refers to the fact that this lock is helpful in bringing Energy up - simplistically stated - the spine. Some schools of thought place this Lock lower down the torso. Not for pregnant women.

Jalandhara Bandha

(Jahl-ahn-dar-ah Bahn-duh). The Chin Lock. This is really a Throat Lock, because that is the area you are locking, not your Chin; but this is the name that has stuck. You take your chin down and your chest up. Okay for pregnant women.

Retention & Suspension

"Inhale" and "Exhale" are self-explanatory. "Retention" in this Guidebook refers to holding the breath after you have Inhaled, ("Antara Kumbhaka"), or at points during your Inhale or Exhale. "Suspension" refers to elongating the space after your Exhale, when there is much less air in the system – thus you are suspending the breath, ("Bahya Kumbhaka").

Note: as you progress in Pranayama the Kumbhakas become more and more important.

Chakra

(Chahk-rah). Chakras are Energy Centers in the body. There is of course conflicting information about their existence, composition and mystical "meanings." In my opinion, based on my personal experience, it is quite appropriate to think of them, at the least, as accessible "power points," though I know them to be more. And to realize that with them you can very much enhance the flow of good Energy, at the least, throughout your physical body.

The Seven Major Chakras

First: Perineum	"Muladhara"	"Root Place"
Second: Low Abdomen	"Swadisthana"	"The Abode of the One"
Third: Solar Plexus	"Manipura"	"City of Gems"
Fourth: Heart	"Anahata"	"Unstruck"
Fifth: Lower Throat	"Visudda"	"Pure"
Sixth: Third Eye	"Ajna"	"Command"
Seventh: Top of Head	"Sahasrara"	"Thousand Petalled Lotus"

It is my belief that each of the Chakra's names have quite instructive meanings. This belief will be discussed at various points in this Guidebook.

How to Get the Most Out of Your Practice

1
Practice Daily

You should try to practice Pranayama as frequently as possible.

Daily is best.

The Basic Truths Behind It

The most important reason why you should practice daily, or very nearly every day, is that Pranayama is a purification, a cleaning-out process. You are, as it were, cleaning out your pipes – (the subtle Energy pipes inside your body) – by… well, let's say by flushing them. A daily flushing through the pipes keeps them clean, and opens you up to flowing in synch with the Universe.

It's the same principle as brushing your teeth every day. If you don't do so, gunk builds up and leads to disease. With Pranayama there's an even bigger reward – Overall Ease versus Dis-Ease. When you do your practice, day after day, then, over time, your life can improve. And you can <u>notice</u> it improving. What a wonderful incentive!

I am <u>not</u> saying that challenges, failures, missteps and setbacks, some even immense and horrendously serious, don't continue to come along.

But when they do, you tend to handle them better. You go through them. They become more instructive, and not as destructive.

A second important, and related, reason to practice often is that daily practice not only keeps you "clean," but also provides you with a maximum cumulative effect. That is, your pipes get purer and purer and purer, just as your gums can get better and better when you floss regularly. Improvement accelerates. You become more and more like clear, flowing water. The "bad" things that happen in your life pass through you, their stains flowing, more easily, away. You find yourself starting to make better decisions. And, happily, this can snowball.

A third reason for regular practice is that, although Pranayama seems simple, there are immense subtleties to it. And you are able to notice these subtleties more when you are able to compare today's practice with yesterday's. And with that knowledge, your skill – your ability to understand and utilize these subtleties in order to go even deeper – grows.

Just as the practiced eye of an experienced Yoga Teacher is able to pick out the subtle workings of a student's body in a Yoga pose, you become more sensitized to, and more able to pick up on, the nuances of the various Pranayama.

Don't Beat Yourself Up if You Miss a Few Days

Pranayama will still be there waiting for you. And notice, when you start again, how much your system loves it. In that way a Pranayama practice is very much like an Asana practice: the more your body experiences it, the more it seems to crave it.

2
Practice in the Early Morning

The Basic Truths Behind It

First of all, you are going to be working with Energy in your lower body. It is therefore best for you to have an empty stomach, bladder and colon when you do your practice.

I cannot overemphasize how much fullness in the abdomen can impede your ability to do the Pranayama practices described here.

And – this being the case – the best time in your day to most easily achieve these conditions is most likely to be just after you get up.

Secondly, if you practice first thing, the demands of the day cannot squeeze the practice out of your schedule. There is always something "more important" or "more immediate" during the days. And then at night, well, you may tend to be "just too tired."

Food in Your Belly

Even a partially-filled stomach can get in your way. I myself, for example, can't eat even one small energy bar and then practice successfully immediately afterwards.

Note that I am not saying that you cannot practice Pranayama with food in your belly, just that the practice will not be anywhere near as effective. This is an important consideration.

> Fullness in your belly inhibits your breathing.

Having eaten also tends to create distractions. You may get tummy gurgling, even during your more static practices, or burp up food, or have gas, or have the taste of your meal still infusing your breath, or have your throat feel constricted by the residue of the food that has passed down it. All these are distractions that are best avoided.

Being too close in time to your last meal will also make it difficult for you to physically work the belly around as you need to do in many of the Pranayama.

If you do eat a small meal – say for example a 200 calorie energy bar and some liquid – I suggest that you wait an hour before practicing.

Some Guidebooks recommend...

> (Note: "Guidebooks" rather than "Sacred Texts" or "Yogic Scriptures." Who cares if something was written 2,000 years ago or yesterday? Or if it was written by someone in the Indus Valley or in Silicon Valley? Again: does Your Own Experience confirm it?)

Some Guidebooks recommend Pranayama at dawn or dusk, or both. Or both of these and at noon and at midnight. Assuming, however, that you have a life to live, and/or are fond of sleep, the pre-dawn, right after getting up, is a superb time for Pranayama – even if you might not agree with the Guidebooks' "balance of lunar and solar energies" theory concerning the equality of both your external environment and your nostrils at these times, and the resultant beneficial "centralization."

PRACTICE IN THE EARLY MORNING

Some reasons for having an early morning practice:

> The noises of the day do not intrude. No one else is stirring about, disrupting.
>
> Digestion does not interfere with your Meditation.
>
> You have not just had some great big emotional experience that gets in your way. As in "I'm so excited I can't sit down." (Best not to check your communications before practicing, as information received may grab at your mind or emotions.)
>
> On a related note, later in the day the mind may be more buzzy from the adventures of the day and may need a lot more time to settle down.
>
> Studies show that people who do things early in the morning tend to stick with them.
>
> The darkness is calming. Your eyes have to work – <u>even when they are shut</u> – when there is any light at all, natural or artificial. (If you practice in daylight a curtained room would be a good idea.)
>
> Darkness insures that any internal light phenomena you experience are actually being generated inside you rather than being influenced by some outer source.
>
> It is absolutely essential to be well-rested, to achieve concentration.
>
> It is best to be both empowered and at peace, sexually, to be balanced. And in my opinion this is the best time of the day to achieve that.
>
> <u>It is a most wonderful way to start your morning</u>.

Need some "early-bird' incentive? How about this:

This Is the
MOST IMPORTANT THING
You Will Do All Day

so...

MAKE TIME!

Don't think that you are too rushed to practice in the morning. If you want anything enough you can craft a way to make it happen. You'll find time, somewhere, for it.

Or, rephrasing this as an unpleasant "tough love" reality: if you can't find a way to do something, you may think you want it, but you don't really want it.

I myself get up very early in order to be able to do my practice before dawn. For years I have bounced around, usually rising, depending on the obligations of my daily life, between 3:00 AM and 4:30 AM. I now actually feel guilty if I sleep in past 4:30.

I am more than willing to get up this early because I have found that it is the best way for me to insure that I do my Pranayama. Years ago I would have thought that rising so early was extreme. Now it just seems normal to me. In fact I am so habituated to it that I usually wake up just before the alarm rings.

I am, however, only able to do this because my daily schedule allows me to go to bed quite early and get a good night's sleep. And because I can also get further rest and refreshment during the day: in my seventeen-minute Perfection Period during my Pranayama session; and perhaps in an hour-long Yoga Nidra/Japa session, or in a mid-day Siesta, or by logging in one or two twenty-minute "Power Naps."

Of course I am not recommending that you get up so early tomorrow morning, or ever. This is just what I personally have found optimal. You are not a bad person if you don't get up before the crack of dawn to do Pranayama.

My point is that you might want to find some way to make an early morning time available to you. Maybe get up a quarter-hour or half-hour earlier, at the start, if necessary, in order to make time. Then see how things progress.

Yes, getting out of a warm bed early is a hard thing to do, but doing it consistently – slashing through the "Gordian Knot" difficulty of it – gives you a marvelous sense of empowerment that I think is well worth cultivating. You become more content with yourself. Doing it each day becomes a matter of self-respect.

So, a hint. It is very helpful to train yourself to kick your covers off and swing your legs out of bed at the very first ring of your alarm clock. Getting the covers off is half the battle; swinging the legs and sitting up is the other half.

The first month or so is the hardest. The good news is that after that it becomes a bit harder _not_ to swing your legs out of the bed and sit up. And, once sitting up, it's easier:

Stand up…

Walk away from the bed…

Don't look back…

And look at things this way: having won this battle…the rest of the day should be a piece of cake.

SQUEEZE THE DAY!

Sorry. I got carried away.

Temperature & Noise

As a related aside: I myself have good results in a room with the temperature at 65 degrees Fahrenheit. But I like cool temperatures and dislike heat. Find the temperature that works for you, and try to have the temperature set up before you begin your practice.

Keep in mind that you will be lying down in your Perfecting phase, and to maximize the potency of that phase your feet and your hands should not be feeling cold. In my opinion, your feet can be covered during Perfection but your hands might be best left open to the air.

An air conditioner or heater that is making noise or blowing air can be a distraction. I have experimented, however, with background noises during my sessions, to try to test and enhance my concentration abilities, and have found that one can practice successfully despite them. "Stillness in the Heart of Action."

Or... Practice Any Time

Okay. Yes, I personally think the early morning is a wonderful time to practice, and I am not alone in that opinion.

That said, it is more important to get a practice in than to obsess about an iron-clad schedule; most important to practice, whatever the timing.

3
Clean Your Systems

The Basic Truth Behind It

For your Pranayama to be most potent you need to have a wide-awake body and mind, and to also have clean and unobstructed respiratory and elimination systems. Any obstruction impinges upon, or even blocks, your abilities.

The abdomen, especially, can impinge on the breath. And the abdomen also needs to be open so that Energy can flow.

A Suggested Preparation Sequence

With all that in mind, this chapter sets out a possible preparation sequence (for an early morning practice) that you may find helpful. Its suggestions are not <u>essential</u>. What is essential is to find a way to the end result – a body and mind ready to sit and concentrate without any internal distractions.

<u>RPM.</u> Karen B., a meditation instructor, passed a tip on to me that pares morning pre-practice preparation down to an absolute minimum. Karen practices and teaches "RPM" – "Rise, Pee, Meditate."

My normal preparation sequence, though, adds a few more of what I consider to be beneficial activities: I rise, and promptly (1) pee, and possibly defecate, (2) take a quick hot shower and then dunk myself twice in a tub of cold water, (3) brush my teeth and scrape my tongue, (4) clean my nostrils and sinuses with a neti pot, (5) dress, (6) feed the cat, sigh, (7) have a couple swallows of a coffee/coconut water mix, (and, if my urine was dark, I also have a few ounces of water), and (8) do a brief headstand-type inversion.

This preparation is quick and effective: thirty to forty minutes after my alarm rings, I am sitting down in my chair and beginning my Pranayama session.

I feel that this kind of preparation sequence can work quite satisfactorily for you, but only if you are fully rested and your respiratory and elimination systems are clear. If you are not fully rested it might be better to wait until you have been up longer and feel more wide awake. And if there is congestion in your respiratory and/or elimination systems you should wait and deal with it.

I will now explain the reasoning behind five of the activities I do, as listed above.

(1) Voiding the Bladder and Colon

For good results in Pranayama you need an empty lower body.

You are working with air, with Energy, and with both Energetic and physical movement, in your lower abdomen. A full bladder or a full colon will very much impede your ability to do so.

To experience the truth of this statement, the next time you sit down on the toilet to defecate, try churning your stomach around and/or doing quick deep Inhales and/or leaning forward and down and twisting to the side. Notice the obvious connection between your physical actions and the movement of feces.

I repeat: you cannot practice successfully on a full bladder or a full colon. If you haven't voided your <u>bladder</u> prior to Pranayama you will feel impeded in your very first Pranayama. Thus you should urinate when you get up. (A cold shower can help bring about a more complete emptying of the bladder.)

Likewise, fullness in your <u>colon</u> will not only impede your ability to do the Pranayama, it will impede the efficacy of your Perfecting phase, after you have completed your active Pranayama. And, on a broader level, a system with a lot of feces in it will tend to make you feel both physically and mentally loggy and disinclined.

(2) Taking a Hot-Cold Shower/Cold Bath

Just a few minutes after having left your seductively soft, warm bed, dunking yourself a few times in a cold tub, (or, if you like, taking a cold shower), will leave you <u>WIDE AWAKE</u>. And this is important. You do not want to be at all sleepy: you are going to sit, completely stationary, for a long period of time.

I shower first, running warm or hot water all over my body for a minute or so. Why? Because my body likes it, and it seems to somehow set me up for the cold blast that follows.

There are two other Pranayama-related reasons for this shower.

(1) Steam and hot water furthers nasal and colonic cleansing – hot water helps urge any remaining feces out. (And the cold tub-water will help clench out any remaining urine.)

(2) Body odor can be a distraction. (As can the smell of lotion if you put it on your body after your shower.)

Well, maybe there's another benefit. I have not quantified this but I currently believe that we might well be more open to the benefits of Pranayama when we are not carrying around any Energetic baggage. Just as the Japanese leave their shoes at the door and thus perhaps do not bring outside Energy into the tranquility of their homes, so we may be better off ridding our bodies of some of our accumulated Energies.

Because of the dramatic effect that a hot, steamy shower has in opening up your respiratory systems, and the dramatic wakefulness that my hot/cold sequence brings about, my opinion – based on years and years of experience – is that some sort of shower and/or tub sequence like this is a very, very good preparation for you if you wish to obtain the <u>full</u> benefits of an early morning Pranayama practice.

You can of course clean yourself with soap in the shower, under the warm water, first, before going into your cold water regimen. I do not, because I take a cleansing shower later in the morning, after exercise.

Aside from Pranayama considerations, my Hot Shower/Cold Tub sequence leaves me feeling both wonderful and invigorated. I have come to think of it as a potent form of hydrotherapy, leading to better health. I've even learned to enjoy the process. I think of it as the equivalent of the Norse practice of a hot sauna followed by a jump into an icy lake. There must be a reason my Swedish ancestors did that. And again: anything, if made habit, becomes, over time, natural and normal.

<u>Note on a Side Benefit of Pranayama</u>

Nowadays I do not need a cold shower/tub-dunk in order to wake up <u>mentally</u>. One apparent result of doing a regular, lengthy Pranayama practice is that I ordinarily wake up each morning with a completely clear <u>head</u>.

(My pre-cold-water <u>body</u> on the other hand…)

This has been something totally new for me – previously in my life I would have experienced, even after a very long sleep, varying degrees of grogginess upon awakening. I felt, as I suspect most of us do, that this was normal. But I now feel very much like a light bulb that goes instantly from OFF – "CLICK!" – to complete ON, to full brightness, as soon as I open my eyes, swing my legs out of bed and sit up. This "on-in-an-instant" feeling is wonderful; my head and brain feel clear and light. I never cease to marvel over it.

(3) Cleaning the Mouth

Why <u>emphasize</u> a clean mouth for Pranayama? Because you breathe in and out through the mouth in some of the Pranayama, and in others its status affects the breath.

Brushing your Teeth

This is a good idea if your mouth does not feel fresh when you wake, (and whose does?). I suggest however using just a dab of toothpaste, if that. Using too much toothpaste can lead to distracting tastes and smells during Pranayama. I myself do not use any toothpaste at this early morning point in my day. Besides my teeth, I also brush the roof of my mouth, inner cheeks and underneath my tongue. Most of the bacteria in the mouth are on the tongue and inner cheeks.

Scraping your Tongue

I use a purpose-built plastic scraper to scrape the top of my tongue, especially the rear of the tongue, scraping it lightly five or six times in quick succession. Why? Notice the amount and color of the gunk, gunk that your toothbrush doesn't get.

Some tongue scrapers are metal. I've used both kinds. I don't feel any lack using plastic.

Option: Flossing and/or Gargling

You might want to consider one or both of these. I don't consider them essential for Pranayama, but as much purity in the mouth as possible cannot hurt.

But if you do gargle, I suggest you do so with an extremely watered-down mouthwash. I've found gargling with normal strength mouthwash can lead – like using too much toothpaste – to excessive swallowing and throat tightness during Pranayama.

Further, over-gargling in the back of the mouth/upper throat may disguise any "Amrita/Soma Center" perfume you may be fortunate enough to generate during your Pranayama.

I myself wait until after my breakfast to floss and gargle.

(4) Neti Pot Cleaning

Neti Pot Cleaning ("Jal Neti" or "Jala Neti") is the process of pouring tepid, slightly salted water into one nostril and letting it flow out the other. This opens up your nasal passages and thus very much enhances your Pranayama. And – Pranayama aside – using a Neti Pot cleans the upper respiratory system for better breathing during the day, and helps prevent respiratory ailments.

Using a Neti Pot will be discussed in more detail in Volume II.

(8) Doing a Brief Inversion

This is <u>NOT</u> for Beginners. I will discuss it more in Volume II.

I myself do not do a regular headstand; I go upside-down for five minutes in a headstand-type apparatus sold by Gaiam. I do this, in part, because I am concerned about the dangers of spinal disc compression so soon after rising.

The combination of Neti Pot cleaning followed by upside-downing brings a much welcome and useful openness and purity to the breath.

A Vigorous-Exercise Alternative

An alternative sequence for those who wish to exercise immediately upon rising can also work well. After having peed and/or defecated, ten minutes of vigorous full-body exercise will wake you up and clear out your respiratory channels, and thus very much enable your Pranayama.

You can then go on with the rest of my previously-discussed suggested sequence if you wish.

Preparation Sequence: The Essence

I have just spent a lot of time discussing pre-practice regimens. I have done so because doing these few basic preparations has proven to be a most effective way for me to set myself up for success in my early morning Pranayama session – and, even further, because over the years I have come to firmly believe that each portion of the preparation adds to the potency of my session.

And not only do I consider doing these things to be a useful purification process, I always feel good after having completed them.

I myself have followed regimens of this sort for years. But, again, look for the essence of what I am relating. Find <u>your</u> optimal preparation for the lengthy period of sitting and breathing into which you are about to put yourself.

And again, I feel the essence is this:

> Your body and your mind must be
> wide awake
> calm
> unobstructed

4

Calm Your Belly

The Basic Truth Behind It

A hungry stomach is a huge distraction during Pranayama and Meditation. You <u>must</u> therefore take steps to prevent this distraction. You <u>must</u> <u>not</u> become hungry during your practice.

If, as I suggest, you practice in the early morning, prior to breakfast, I think it is however a very good idea to put <u>something</u> in your stomach.

This is the seventh step of my early-morning pre-practice regimen that was discussed in the previous chapter.

Quiet the Hunger in Your Stomach

What works for me quite well is a very small amount of cold liquid – half cold coffee and half coconut water.

Over time I've discovered that one mouthful - two swallows - of this mixture is my maximum. Anything more than that and the mix tends to slosh around in my stomach during Pranayama, or get in the way of the belly–related practices, or may make my throat raspy.

I do not usually sip water because I like the mental alertness I feel I get with coffee.

However – though I suspect that the coffee gives me a better mental edge, a better concentration in Pranayama and Meditation, and also believe that it makes me much less prone to lose concentration or even (horror of horrors) doze off – I have found that anything more than this amount of coffee tends to make my brain <u>too</u> active during both of these practices.

It took me years to discover the coffee/coconut water blend. Tea proved to be somehow too harsh on the respiratory system for me. Orange juice, milk, soy milk or cocoa didn't work. <u>Hot</u> coffee mixed with milk tended to close down my throat during Pranayama, to make it catchy and feel too full of phlegm, and thus force me to swallow time after time to try to free things up. Butter in milk led to nausea after belly/breath work. And note well: the currently-marketed "energy drinks" do NOT work.

I drink this before my headstand because I want the fluid in the belly to start being absorbed before I sit down to practice.

<u>Water for Dehydration.</u> If your morning urine is dark yellow it means you are dehydrated. This is not an optimal state to be in for Pranayama – or for anything else, for that matter. This occurs only rarely with me, but when it does I also drink 4-6 ounces of room-temperature water, with a bit of lemon juice squeezed into it. This does not seem to overly impede my practice.

Why not Solid Food?

Because it doesn't leave your stomach as quickly as liquid. And too, little bits of it may still remain inside your mouth, a distraction as you practice.

A Final Note on these Preliminaries

All this getting ready - my morning toilet, dressing, etc. - takes me 30 to 40 minutes.

Thus, with <u>focus</u> and <u>economy of action</u>, I can do all this and be on my chair, beginning my Pranayama, with my body and mind absolutely wide awake, in the early morning darkness, as early as 3:30.

This focus and economy of action took discipline at first, but, again, flowed easily once habitual.

One important hint is to set <u>everything</u> up the night before. Then you can just breeze, unthinking, through the sequence.

And further, I suggest setting things up in the <u>early</u> evening; you may well find that you get "just too tired" later in the evening.

5

Wear Helpful Clothing

The Basic Truth Behind It

You need to wear non-constricting clothing. Your chest, belly and arms need to be able to move freely. And you need to be able to sit without feeling excessively hot or cold.

Recommended Clothing

In my opinion, a tee shirt and shorts work very well. Make sure your tee shirt is loose everywhere, not tucked in. You don't want to constrict the body, especially the movement of the belly.

Shorts might be best because you'd like your forearms and wrists to rest solidly on your thighs – skin-on-skin – rather than possibly slipping on the fabric of pants or leotards. A short-sleeve shirt may thus also be more useful than a long-sleeve shirt.

That said, a long-sleeve shirt and long pants that are both made of a non-slippery fabric can, if loose around the tummy, torso and arms, work very well.

Wear cool clothes rather than hot – you will most probably heat up from your breathing, and you might even become sweaty. All-Cotton has worked well for me, and it isn't clingy. That said, I have not noticed any deleterious effects from wearing synthetics.

I have experimented with various clothing colors but have not as yet been able to definitively identify differing results. I have had superb results with both light gray clothing and black, as well as with "synthetic" and "natural" clothes.

In a similar vein, I have not yet quantified whether there is a difference when I wear absolutely clean clothing (i.e., allegedly "Energy-neutral") as opposed to previously-worn clothing (i.e., allegedly carrying some sort of Energetic impact). From my experiences I <u>suspect</u> there is some difference.

Your Groin

Sometimes dampness will accumulate in the groin from the intensity of your practice. I myself am, most often, unaware of the dampness <u>during</u> my practice; it does not usually intrude. But, previously, I have had on many occasions to change into another jock strap, and sometimes even new shorts – because of the amount of dampness accumulated – when I got up from my chair to lie down on my couch for my Perfecting phase.

So, because of this possibility of dampness, though I used to wear elasticized Yoga shorts, I no longer do so. I wear loose shorts in order to aerate my groin area more fully.

Your Feet

Your feet must not be cold; it's an immense distraction if they are. I suggest that at the least you wear socks, if needed. I myself wear socks and – gasp – shoes. Not only for foot warmth in the cold morning but also for leg/torso stability, (the shoes anchor my feet into the floor). Note that I am sitting in a chair, not on the floor.

Options

On cold mornings I may wear a light vest-jacket over my tee shirt. I can unzip the vest or even slip it off as I warm up during my Pranayama.

And/or, on really cold mornings, I may drape a Tibetan-yak-wool shawl, gifted to me by two of my students, Patty and Anna Maria, over my shoulders, (or wrap it around my bare legs). The advantage of a "prayer shawl" like this is that it can be easily sloughed off, by degrees if you wish, as your body heats up from doing your Pranayama. On cold days you can keep your hands tolerably warm under it, or at other times they can peek out.

6

Practice for a Set Time Period

The Basic Truth Behind It

You need to commit yourself, when you sit down for Pranayama, to sitting there for a <u>set period of time</u>.

This is because Pranayama can be, initially, Boring. It is therefore quite likely that you may not stay with it, at first, without artificial assistance:

> "I'm bored. I'm just sitting here breathing. Nothing's happening... Oh, to hell with it, I'm getting out of here."

With time, however, Pranayama becomes Fascinating. Before that happens, though, you should commit to your practice, on the grounds that you know that, (as happens with an Asana practice), you will feel really, really good once you do start, and that afterwards you will consistently feel, besides all the other benefits, an enormous, quiet satisfaction.

"Getting" Pranayama

Some beginning Pranayama students come up to me and say, "Tom, I just don't get it." And they don't. Because it takes consistent practice over time for Pranayama to take hold.

Pranayama is not a quick, easy fix. It is learned behavior. You mustn't think that, just because it is as simple as sitting there and breathing, it's simple. It's not. It requires work, dedication, patience.

If that prospect is overly daunting to you, you may not be ready for a Pranayama practice. That's okay. You may want to practice Asana for some period of time in order to open yourself to Pranayama.

Indeed, some schools of Yogic thought do not encourage the introduction of Pranayama until the student has been adequately versed in Asana. This is based, at least in part, on the belief that Asana is necessary to sufficiently prepare the body's Energy channels.

My experience has been that those students in my classes who do have an Asana and/or Meditation background are, generally, much more likely to "get" Pranayama, quickly.

Set a Timer

I think the best way to make sure that you stay "in" for a set period of time, day after day, week after week, etc., is to set a timer and commit yourself to just sitting there doing your Yogic Breathing, or – if it comes to that – just sitting there, breathing – until it pings.

But by all means don't be locked in by your timer. Keep on going after it pings, if the spirit moves you. (Yoga Joke.)

I Just Don't *Feel* Like It!

Sometimes, or often, for various reasons, you will not feel like doing your Pranayama practice on any given day, even though rationally you know that it is in your best interest to do so.

PRACTICE FOR A SET TIME PERIOD

One way to overcome this block is to trick yourself into practicing. You can start by just setting a timer for a short period of time, (maybe just five minutes or so), and promising yourself that you will just sit there for that period of time. "I'll just do that, and then I'll get up and go about my day. *Anybody* can just sit for five minutes."

Hopefully this "just sitting" period will induce an initial calming down and bring about a change in your emotional state, so that you will actually want to continue sitting there, and will add some Pranayama to your sitting.

And if the Pranayama itself also takes you further "in," you might find that you may also just want to sit there afterwards – just sitting there in a meditative posture for some minutes after the end of your "active Pranayama."

This trickery is a great example of how just sitting quietly – and especially just sitting there and getting in touch with your breath – can change your emotional state, your mood, right around. So that you then very much "feel like it."

If it doesn't work – if you just can't seem to get started: okay, just sit there for a while. You are helping to building up the habit. And you have managed to salvage something for your self-esteem: "Well, at least I sat!"

My Personal Practice

For my current practice I usually set three timers:

(1) One for, usually, 45 minutes or less, for my settling in and active Pranayama.

(2) A second, usually for 10-15 minutes, for the meditative "Sitting" period that follows the active Pranayama.

I am currently sometimes prone to dedicating this period to a potent Energetic practice called Bija Mantra, which will be discussed in Volume II, or to a more advanced practice which I call Long Distance Partner

Work, (to be discussed in Volume III), or a combination of the two. If however I am doing types of these practices with other practitioners later in the day I might merely Sit without – I admit it – any timer at all.

(3) A third for exactly 17 minutes, for my lying-down "Perfecting" period that follows my Sitting.

Yes, that's a practice that lasts well over an hour. But I am by no means suggesting to you that you practice that long. It took me years and years to arrive at that length of time.

And though these lengths of time are not arbitrary and have solidified over time because they have proven to be an effective template for me, I am not a slave to them.

Previously I would occasionally do even longer times, but I have come to consider 45 minutes of "active" practice a good maximum for me, because:

1. It allows me to get several of the active Pranayama into my session if I wish to do so.
2. It gives me ample time to explore something in depth if I am led into directions that seem promising;
3. I have come to feel that I get diminishing returns after that approximate time frame.

Sometimes, sigh, my 45-minute timer goes off but I still want to "stay in" and work more. It takes discipline to come out at that time.

Other Yoga Teachers (Broadly) Concur

Regarding doing a practice of the length that I do: I do not consider it coincidental that the well-regarded Yoga Teacher B.K.S. Iyengar concurs: "Set aside 40-60 minutes at a fixed time of day for the pranayama." Yoga: The Path To Holistic Health, page 231.

Further, Yogani – an experienced, contemporary Yoga Teacher – also recommends, for an advanced morning practice, seventy-five minutes. And Yogani divides the session up into three sections: Pranayama, Meditation and Resting, which correlate perfectly – it's just a matter of the verbiage – with my Pranayama, Sitting and Perfection phases.

PRACTICE FOR A SET TIME PERIOD

Sidetrack: Yogani

"Yogani" is the pseudonym of a Yogi in Florida who has written several bite-size books (and one big, encompassing book titled <u>Advanced Yoga Practices</u>). He has also set up websites. His aim is to offer us a deceptively simple yet deeply effective Pranayama / Meditation practice. In doing so he discusses a full gamut of Yogic theory, including a cursory discussion of Asana.

Though his system differs from what is offered here, Yogani's discoveries and discussions resonate well with my experiences. And, as far out as some of his thinking first appeared to me, I find myself so very often meeting him – as they say — as he is coming back down the mountain.

How Long is Right for You?

All well and good. But what I advise <u>you</u> to do first is to discover a shorter length of time that works for you initially. Perhaps <u>fifteen minutes</u>. Iyengar states, with an unexplained assertiveness, that "a minimum of fifteen minutes a day is essential." <u>Light on Pranayama</u>, page 55.

Twenty to thirty minutes should work. If for some reason I am pressed for time in the morning I can cut my practice down to that.

I do not think you can practice for less than 10 minutes on a regular basis and still make good progress. Thus I think it best to think of a 5-minute practice as merely a Quickie, useful for travel or rushed situations, or for any time you just want to take a short break and quiet down – but not as something that is appropriate for your "regular practice," the practice that you need in order to develop Pranayama's full power.

Otherwise, when you only have five minutes: Meditate.

I am further of the opinion, formed from experience, that a Sitting Step needs to last at least five minutes in order to be effective. And that a Perfection Step should last at least ten minutes.

So – if you do have a half hour you might try dividing it up between a fifteen-minute settling in and active Pranayama session, five minutes of Sitting and ten minutes of lying down in Perfection.

Whatever length of time you choose, I strongly believe you <u>need</u> to end your session with this "Perfecting" period, for recovery and curing and… well… Perfecting.

Use Trial and Error

But again, my suggestions are just suggestions, not fiat. Find out for yourself, as always through trial and error, a time or times that work for you.

When you find a promising length of time, <u>Stick To It</u> for a good while. Give it time to take hold and become habitual. And then see if, over time, you grow to want even more time "inside." I think you might.

And note that if you become completely engaged in the practice, (as you should be), you can become so fascinated by and caught up in what is occurring that time loses its meaning. My active Pranayama portion often seems to go by in the blink of an eye; sometimes it shocks the hell out of me when my timer pings.

How to Settle In

Before you begin what I call your "active" Pranayama – the breathwork in which you Inhale and Exhale and Retain and Suspend in various combinations – it is important to become as calm and focused as possible.

Rather than just plunk yourself down and jump right into doing all the various Pranayama, it is much better to settle in and allow the practice to come to you.

These next three chapters are designed to be helpful in that regard.

7

How to Use External Posture

The Basic Truths Behind It

You want to "lose" your body so that you can concentrate. You want to make it "disappear." To do so, your posture must be comfortable and stable.

Your spine should be erect, to enhance proper Energy Flow.

The Three Main Things

1. **Be comfortable**. This is necessary so that you are not in any way distracted by any difficulties in the body and can concentrate on your Breathing and Meditation.
2. **Be stable**. This is necessary in order to quiet down both the body and the mind. If you feel a need to wiggle around or fidget about you get distracted. So you want to find a (comfortable) position for your body that you can stay in, and then stay in it. Body movement

begets thinking. (The flip side: mental distractions can make you physically fidgety. It's all mind-body, body-mind.)

My understanding is that these two requirements are in fact the very first directives about Yogic sitting contained in the ancient Yogic text, the Yoga Sutras. The translation of Sutra 2:46 – "sthira sukham asanam" – that I like best is:

> "The asana is a position of comfort and stability."
> <u>Raja Yoga Pranayama</u>, G. Gautama, p. 18
> (With thanks to A. Ran)

3. **Be Upright**. To <u>fully</u> benefit from Pranayama it is essential to have an upright spine (at the least up to the neck), rather than a slouchy posture. This is so that your breath and, primarily, the Energy in your body can flow. Don't Slouch!

Being upright does not mean losing the natural curves of your spine.

Cross-Legged Floor-Sitting

Yogic cross-legged floor-sitting poses can work very well for Pranayama. They are designed to do so. But I do not recommend them for beginning or intermediate practitioners for several reasons.

First, most of us lifelong-chair-sitting Westerners cannot hold ourselves up for a long period of time sitting cross-legged and straight up without our backs getting in our way. We start to ache, or we slouch, or both. I have noticed this even with the students in my advanced Yoga classes, and with the supposedly more advanced practitioners in Yoga teacher training groups. Most everyone ends up, after a while, slouchy, slithery and comfy.

A second reason not to sit cross-legged on a floor is that – unless you are very open in the hips – your knees will be raised up off the floor. This leads to instability. And it is important for your knees to be at least as low as your hips, (even lower than the hips can be better), so as to not close down your abdomen and chest, and to help in creating an erect spine.

Sitting on a Meditation cushion works well to achieve this, but only if you are comfortable and stable, and with your knees on the floor (or at least slightly lower than the hips and perhaps supported by blankets or foam blocks).

A third reason not to sit cross-legged is that your legs tend to become numb as you sit. I have even seen the feet of advanced students turning blue as they sat there, adamantly cross-legged. Moreover, when these advanced students come out of the floor-seated portion of their Pranayama session in order to lie down in their Perfecting phase, they will most often get all tingly in the legs, or experience other discomfort, and will have to wriggle about, stretch or even massage their legs – which of course completely disrupts the necessary stillness of the Perfecting period, and takes them right out of this important phase.

In an effort to avoid these things, many floor-sitting students will change the cross of their legs every so often as they sit there. This is an unfortunate distraction. Nevertheless – trying to make the best of it – I tell students in my classes and workshops to go ahead and change the cross of their legs every once in a while during our Pranayama session if they wish to, but to make sure they do it when they are in-between individual Pranayama.

I think this inability to sit cross-legged comfortably and with stability is mostly caused by our having sat in chairs from year one. And perhaps we may not have the requisite core strength. But whatever the reason, this inability is where most all of the people I see are at. And I think therefore we should adapt accordingly: too many relatively-new-to-Yoga students who attend my classes or workshops seem to feel they must sit on the floor, because that is "Yoga." Or because they let their egos get in the way, and try to match the more advanced students, to (as always in Yoga) their detriment.

I will address these postures more in Volume III.

Using a Meditation Bench

One less stressful alternative to cross-legged sitting, for those physically able, is to sit on the floor, on your heels, with your buttocks on a meditation bench and your knees close together.

In Yoga this is called the "Vajrasana" pose. It is a good posture for Pranayama and Meditation because you may be able to hold it comfortably for long period and because it helps you to keep your spine in its erect position without the distraction of excessive muscular effort.

I utilize a meditation bench most often during partner or group practices when I want to be seated on the floor at the same level as the other practitioners and wish to stay there for a very long period of time.

I will discuss this option more thoroughly in Volume II.

Chair/Sofa Sitting

I personally think the vast majority of readers of this book – including those who haven't had years and years of Asana experience that may possibly have opened their hips – might be best served by doing the practice seated on a chair or sofa rather than a floor. And so, because I would like the life-enhancing practices in this Guidebook to be available for use by the widest possible audience, most all that follows is directed to a practitioner sitting in a chair.

Why on earth should the marvelous benefits of Pranayama be confined to only those among us with open hips?

The good news is that sitting on a couch or a sofa works fine. Sitting in a relatively rigid chair with a back is even better, because its rigidity helps you sit up straighter.

I myself often sit on a metal folding chair with a padded seat and back. Any supportive chair that allows you to sit up straight should work. But note that on chairs with arms the chair arms can get in the way.

(I used to sit a an unpadded metal folding chair with a folded Yoga mat on top of the chair seat to give my buttocks solid purchase rather than have them sliding about.)

An Erect Spine

B.K.S. Iyengar, in <u>Light on Yoga</u>, page 432, lists a few floor-sitting postures appropriate for Pranayama, and then states: "Any other sitting posture may be taken provided that the back is kept absolutely erect from the base of the spine to the neck and perpendicular to the floor."

So. "Any other sitting posture" would include sitting in a chair.

Note Iyengar's emphasis on being absolutely erect. For many years, as I sat on my folding chair, I leaned backwards slightly, into the back of it, in order to be able to stay there seated, stable and comfortable for a long period time.

With the passage of years, however, my core – my back and abdominal muscles – became stronger and I became able to sit upright in the chair, for, eventually, well over an hour. This is very, very helpful. Sitting absolutely erect, (but, once again, with your spine in its natural curves), is – as Iyengar instructs – <u>best</u>.

So, yet again Note Well: you will not experience the fuller powers of Pranayama unless you can sit up straight during your practices.

But, as it is a learned skill, one which comes with the development of core strength and perhaps with hip opening, beginners may find it impossible.

So, if you are sitting for an extended period of time, and your core lacks the requisite strength to remain absolutely erect all the way through things, you might try leaning slightly back against the back of your chair, like I used to do, for some or even most of the time, rather than being <u>absolutely</u> straight up and down.

And personally… I do not <u>overly</u> chastise myself if on occasion I do decide to take a bit of a rest and lean slightly back into the back of my chair for a while.

The Ability to Sit with an Erect Spine

To increase your ability to sit straight up for an extended period of time you might wish to try to strengthen your core – the muscles in the front, sides and back of your torso – through targeted exercise. (And through Pranayama.)

I personally have found exercises or weightlifts like "squats" and "deadlifts" and "back extensions" to be especially helpful in increasing lower back strength, but you need to be cautious. It is easy to injure your low back. And I feel the core exercises called Plank and Side Plank are also extremely helpful.

I have spent some time on posture.
It's that important.
Find a posture you can lose yourself in.

8
How to Get Quiet

The Basic Truth Behind It

In order to concentrate on your breathing you need to let go of your everyday concerns and anxieties. You need to lose your body. You need to calm your breath. You need to stop your mind from zinging around.

You quiet your body by sitting.

You quiet your breath by slow breathing.

You quiet your mind by repeating a Mantra.

Eventually you want to be able to slip in and out of a "meditative" or "alternate" state as easily as a fish jumps in and out of water. But you should be content at the start with building towards that goal.

In any event: you want to settle down in order to be able to give the Pranayama your full attention. You need this. You want to be engaged as fully as possible in each and every breath.

Quiet Your Body by Sitting

Just sit quietly for a minute or two, or more. Don't try to do anything at all. Just let the body settle down by itself. In fact you might want to, or need to, just sit there for <u>several minutes</u>.

I am convinced that for optimal results in your practice you need this little settling-in hiatus between "real life" and the beginning of any active Pranayama work. You can't just dive in. You need to let yourself settle. Your upper torso and head, especially, often seem to be "buzzy" or "flighty" when you first sit down. You need instead to get "sinky." To settle your Energies.

The mind seems to need this initial settling-in time in order to work some things out by itself. There most always seem to be some things bubbling beneath the surface of your mind that want to come out and find expression in your conscious mind. And when these have had their moments in the sun, (have been released), it is much easier to settle. So perhaps try settling-in, initially, without using a Mantra, that is without jumping right in and battling to try to keep the mind quiet by repeating a word or phrase over and over.

Many of us have a tendency to want to rush into what we perceive to be the heart of things, i.e., right into doing the "Real Breathing Part," the "Actual Pranayama." Over time, however, an initial quieting down process like this hopefully teaches us patience, and will consequently bring, (also hopefully), some much-needed balance to those of us with go-go-go personalities.

Happily, the body should actually give you a cue when it is ready to proceed into taking your first deep breath. Let it call to you, and perhaps let your first deep breath, as described below, be spontaneous.

Settle/Relax your Body with Oral Exhales

When you are somewhat relaxed from just sitting, you will then almost always benefit from taking one to three Deep Oral Exhales in order to further relax and settle your upper and lower body.

Experiment with the three Exhales described below. See if any or all of them help relax your personal areas of tightness and grip, or help create a nice sense of quieting down. You may feel the need to use one or more of them on any particular day.

FRONT Upper-Body Exhale

Take one deep breath by:

Inhaling through your nose, and then Exhaling long and slow out through your mouth.

Focus on letting this Oral Exhalation quiet and soothe your jaw, throat and sternum. Any or all of this helps bring about a very helpful relaxation. Relaxing the throat is an especially powerful quieter:

> "When the throat is loose and free from contraction the brain is bound to be calm and peaceful."
> Yoga Teacher G.S. Iyengar
> Yoga, A Gem for Women, p 297

Afterwards, take a few more nasal breaths.

REAR Upper-Body Exhale

Inhale again through your nose and Exhale long through your mouth.

This time, however, try to use the Exhale to soften your upper back, your shoulders, and the back of your neck – where so many of us hold much of our tension. Let your shoulders drop.

As you get further into Pranayama and your body purifies, you might be holding less tension in your body and you may thus notice that there is less of a release when you do these two upper body Exhales – because you don't need them as much. But there is bound to be some beneficial release.

Lower-Body Exhale

Again, you Inhale through your nose and Exhale long and slow through your mouth. This time however you can take the Exhale even further down the <u>front</u> of your body, into your upper chest or belly, or, best, all the way down to your genitals, perineum and anus.

As you Exhale let your lower body become heavy and let your sitz-bones become heavier into your chair. This long, slow Exhale can really seat/anchor your sitz-bones.

And even further, and more subtly, for me at least, Exhaling through the mouth like this rather than the nose seems to set the <u>fronts</u> of the sitz-bones a bit better than Exhaling through the nose. If this doesn't work for you, then try for that result with a long <u>nasal</u> Exhale.

Sitting more on the fronts of your sitz-bones is desirable. Ideally after an Exhale like this you should feel like you are more anchored – like a rock even – down into your chair. You can try to focus, session after session, on becoming aware of how solidly you can settle yourself with your Exhale. Over time you might grow in competence at consciously becoming more and more heavy, grounded and solid.

Also, right after this deep breath, (or during your little "do nothing" period before it), might be a good time to scootch around and see whether some changing of your sitting position can help you feel even more solid on your sitz-bones.

A Lower-Body Exhale also helps your spine to arch into a more correct upright position, if you happen to be slouching.

After your Exhale once again take a few more breaths through your nose.

You should find that taking two or three deep Oral Exhales, in some manner like this, relaxes and quiets you down considerably.

In sum: find the areas in which you hold your tensions, and address them.

<u>Preview</u>

Bahya Kumbhaka, (which is discussed in Volume II), is a more advanced quieting Pranayama involving the lower torso. Your Bahya Kumbhaka will flow better when you have done some of these oral Exhales beforehand to relax your torso. The torso is easier, more calm, more compliant.

Quiet Your Breath with Slow Nasal Breathing

Now, breathe calmly in and out a number of times, through your nose.

You may want to begin, once again, by taking a big deep breath in and then letting it out, (but out through the nose this time) – and then go into a series of focused nasal breaths. These do not have to be big and deep. You want to feel relaxed. Do what is most comforting to you.

I strongly suggest that you breathe in and out 10-15 times. I suggest this because I myself almost always do not feel a really nice quieting down kick in before 10 breaths and usually do achieve it by 15.

Calmness in your breath will translate into calmness in your body, just as agitated breathing will induce agitation in the body.

And gradually focus your mind more and more on your breathing, thus quieting your mind also.

Count to Yourself as You Breathe

The mind may not be ready at this point to go into any sort of complicated word-repetition-work (Mantras). It may still be too buzzy. So, as a transition – as something to help you to preliminarily quiet your mind – during these 10-15 breaths you might say to yourself mentally, on your Inhales and Exhales, "oone-oone," "twooo-twooo," "threee-threee," etc. Or, if it seems right to you, you could just count on your Exhales.

I have found that it interrupts my rhythm if I try to say "eleven… eleven" (as well as "thirteen…thirteen," "fourteen …fourteen," and "fifteen… fifteen"), so I substitute another monosyllabic series once I hit ten, thus: "ten…ten, one…one, two…two… …. five…five."

Lengthen Your Exhales

As you breathe, you might after a while want to see if you can gently make your Exhalations <u>longer</u>. Happily, very often this may happen by itself as your breathing makes you more relaxed.

Also see if you can let your sitz-bones become even heavier with at least a few of your Exhales. As your awareness of the subtleties of breathing grows, when you do this Exhalation/sitz-bone sinking you may also feel a subtle opening of the chest and belly, which is helpful.

Become Relaxed, Spacious & Stable

Let your shoulders drop down even further during this process. Notice how you may have been subconsciously holding onto tension in this area. And how you can in fact consciously let go of it.

As you breathe in and out through your nose, the front of your body rises on the Inhale, creating space in the abdomen. And the back of your body goes down on the Exhale, relaxing your chest. You become more balanced.

On an even more subtle level, see if you can also sense how the buttocks subtly spread during your Exhales, helping create a stable "tripod" type of feeling.

"Am I Relaxed? Am I?"

Note: Students actually ask me this.
Note: Yoga is GOOD for these students.

After your 10-15 breaths your body and mind should feel much more calm. The clue that this has happened is that there is a spontaneous lengthening, (perhaps just a little bit), of the space after your Exhale and before your next Inhale. This lengthening puts in a little more relaxation in the breathing process, a few little beats of non-breathing. And this feels good.

So. If the little space after your Exhale grows a little longer, Yes, You are relaxing. Good on you!

Quiet Your Mind with Mantra

With your body and your breath now both calming down, as you continue to breathe quietly, you might try adding the internal repetition of a simple Mantra, (a word or short phrase), for a while.

This is a well-known meditative technique. The mind likes to have something to latch onto in order to quiet itself. But again: in my opinion the mind is not ready at this point, not sufficiently calm and regulated at this point, for the successful repetition of a <u>complex</u> Mantra. And it is almost certainly not ready at this point for "seedless" (i.e., non-focused) Meditation. (And for many of us, might not be so ready for quite some time.)

So. As an example, one Mantra I use is a saying borrowed and adapted from Organized Religion: the delightfully double-edged-sword English translation "The lords are our shepherds, we shall not want."

A bit of a sea change occurred when I switched the wording from "my" and "I" to "our" and "we." And the "our" also forced me to slow down my repetitions in order to clearly enunciate/differentiate between the "our and the preceding "are" – which slowing, happily, helped me to focus more on meaning rather than repetition.

This construct of the saying has proven to be appropriate for me, and has also proven to be an effective lead-in to my version of the next step, ("How to Get Help"). Quite possibly it has been so effective because I know/am convinced I know it to be true.

Note also: this particular saying also flows nicely with my breath; one phrase can be uttered mentally on the Inhale, and the second phrase on the Exhale. Or I can say both phrases on the Inhale <u>and</u> the Exhale, or between the breaths. This ability to synch the Mantra with the breath is important; the Mantra should not get in the way of the breath. The Mantra you choose should be able to synch.

I believe that an extra benefit of repeating a Mantra with spiritual significance, like the kind described above, is that the mind is in some sense purified prior to the start of the active Pranayama. And if such a

Mantra is not done here, then some similar work during the next step, "Getting Help," will serve that purpose. You sometimes come into your session carrying psychological/emotional baggage that you should like to, at the very least, set side for a while in order to achieve optimum results.

OK. In any event: your mind should be <u>soft</u> in order for you to do Pranayama.

Back to Just Breathing

After you have repeated a mantra for a while, or if you realize that your breathing has slowed down considerably, I suggest that you consider letting go of the Mantra and again concentrating on your breath for a while, going back to "oone-oone," "twooo-twooo," "threee-threee," etc. The Mantra has served its initial purpose of calming the mind and inducing even slower breathing, and may possibly now get in the way of your concentration on your breath.

Or you can play back and forth, focusing on your slow breathing and then on your Mantra, letting them enhance each other.

Mantra First: An Alternative Way to Start

The calming sequence discussed above – your body quiets first, and then your breath, and then your mind – is the same as that commonly and effectively used to take students into Savasana ("Corpse Pose") at the end of an Asana class.

There is however an alternative. You may wish to repeat a brief mantra for a while at the very start of your sitting down and settling in period.

This alternative is based on the fact that when, over a period of time, you have linked a particular Mantra with your slow breathing, that Mantra should eventually induce a "Pavlov's Dogs Effect."

The researcher Pavlov rang a bell every time he fed some dogs. After a while the dogs would salivate when the bell was rung, even though no food was offered to them. They had linked the bell to food in their minds.

Similarly, here, repetition of the same Mantra over and over, session after session, as you do your slow breathing, establishes that linkage, and can induce slow rhythmic breathing. The breath hitches a ride on the Mantra.

Because of the Pavlov's Dogs Effect, I strongly suggest that you find, by experimenting over time, the Mantra that best suits you. And then utilize it exclusively, using it in every practice session. Over the weeks, months and years, the Mantra becomes associated not just with slowed breathing but with calmness itself. That is to say, the greater Pavlov's Dogs Effect is that just saying the Mantra to yourself induces calm. This is no small benefit.

I speculate that this may also be one reason why gurus are said to give their students "secret" and "powerful" Mantras for their own personal use. Giving someone something and telling them it is powerful should ensure its continuous use, and being told to keep it a "secret" tends to invest it with even more mystical power.

Note that using your Mantra near the start of your Getting Quiet period can be especially helpful on those occasions when you realize, as you are sitting there at the beginning of your practice, that your mind is particularly buzzy.

Take Whatever Time You Need to Settle

Don't get down on yourself if you do not immediately become immensely quiet and "Yoga-like." I often string out all my preliminaries for as long as fifteen minutes or more before I actually start my active Pranayama. This does not degrade the Pranayama. Not having quieted down, on the other hand, may well do so.

If Phenomena Should Occur

This entire settling-in process may in itself be enough to take you "in" or to put you up into your Third Eye Area or to bring up phenomena. If so, Not to Worry. These are Good Things.

Summation:

Why is "Getting Quiet" an Important First Step?

The more calm and quiet you can become initially the better your Pranayama session should be.

You want to practice your Pranayama in a completely relaxed state so that you are able to practice fully and with the requisite focus.

9

How to Get Help

The Basic Truth Behind It

We <u>need</u> to invoke Assistance. Period. We do not do all this on our own. It flows from grace. I myself would no more go into a Pranayama session without an Invocation than I would go deep sea diving without an oxygen tank.

> **Good Work is that which the people lay claim to Saying**
> **"Amazing! We did it! All by ourselves!"**
>
> <u>Tao Te Chin</u>, Verse 17
> (translations selected by the writer)

Invoke & Internalize a Helper

After your mind has been calmed down sufficiently by your Getting Quiet practices, one way to accomplish this Invocation is to utilize another Mantra (or Mantras) in order to help you <u>internalize</u> Help (or a Helper or Helpers of your choice) according to your spiritual persuasion.

Bring Help to you, with your love, your need and your tremendous intensity.

"Invoke" derives from two Latin words that mean "Call In." Some Indian-based Guidebooks say "Put Guru into your heart." This is not meant figuratively. You may indeed want to use a Mantra to invite Help/Helper(s) which/who are in consonance with your highest aspirations to <u>physically</u> enter your body/heart area and guide you.

Yoga and Religion

Considering the Source of the above suggestion, and indeed of many of my suggestions: Yoga, stripped of its Hindu overlay, (a stripping which does not diminish its potency whatsoever), can be useful whatever Organized Religion or Spiritual Belief you espouse.

Religion/Deep Belief should – in my opinion – reflect essential truth, and Yoga is designed to reveal essential truth. Any persuasion that adamantly turns its back on the postural, breathing or meditative aspects of Yoga is, (again in my opinion), binding itself into itself, perhaps from unfounded fear, and may possibly be rejecting something simply because that something is perceived, perhaps due to ignorance of its true nature, as Alien…is perceived to spring from another Source.

Sidetrack: Namaha & Namaste

> Yoga can be studied, if one wishes, without any bowing down to its Hindu/Indian background. A lot of the "exotic" stuff in Yoga is marketing hype.
>
> I personally, when I teach, honor my Yogic lineage by saying the Indian word "Namaha" at the beginning of my classes, to show that "I bow down to this." (This practice of Yoga.) And by saying "Namaste" to my students at the end of the class, to show them that "I bow down to you."

I use both these terms in order to put myself in my proper place; often a difficult thing for a Teacher as they tend to get more and more used to being obeyed.

But no problem, any way. Yoga is as American as apple pie. It is as English as tea. As Irish as the potato. As Russian as the Cyrillic alphabet. And as Brazilian as, well, Brazil. (There is a, perhaps subtle, point here.)

Invocation as an Opening Ritual

I feel that a ritualized invocation sequence – that is, one which is repeated in exactly the same way each and every time you begin your practice – is a beneficial method with which to open your practice.

A complex invocation, (mine is lengthy), or a simple one, can serve to bring about a helpful daily re-visitation of the "why" of your practice, and, if phrased correctly, can be an equally important daily re-dedication. It can also further your calming.

One Way to Invoke

Do whatever works for you. But whatever you do, make it intense. Just don't internally chant out a recitation. Mean it. You are INVOKING! You are calling, bringing to you, with the intensity of your need. Repetition with Belief!

If you use an Invocation Mantra it can be more complex than one used for quieting the mind.

I myself Invoke and Internalize. I reach out to my Yoga lineage, my backbone. And, with repeated practice at it over years, I became able to sense, first, a difference close by, and then, much later over time, within.

My personal Invocation process creates a very nice feeling. I am enveloped in the love and guidance of my lineage. I am, as it were, being shepherded. And even further: I have been taught about unconditional love.

I do not write the three previous sentences lightly.

You yourself will be able to find something – some Aspect of our Refuge – that gets you there.

Wisdom & Your Invocation

Wisdom has been defined as being able to hold fast to two completely opposite positions. Along those lines, then: it doesn't matter what you construct as long as you know it to be true.

(Is your brain about to explode?)

Moving On

Your Invocation continues the essential settling-in preliminaries, and at the end of it you should feel completely calm and quiet, and foursquare on your own ground.

If you have done your Invocation with the requisite intensity, perhaps now just sit there for a while and take at the least a few more deep breaths before proceeding.

Note that the Getting Help process may also take you "in" a little bit; you may well experience phenomena: head-bobbing, lights, internal levitation, etc., etc. If so, go with it for a while, if you wish, before proceeding. Notice how nice it is:

> **In the arms of the angels**
> **may you find some comfort here**

> from "Angel" by Sarah McLachlin
> [with apologies for changing things]

Thus, armed, proceed.

The Basic Pranayama

Energy-Awakening & Energy-Rising Pranayama

This next group of chapters gives you concepts and practices into which you can dig deeper and deeper, and utilize beneficially, for years and years. Plus it gives you foundational knowledge about Breath and Energy, and why we work them, and how.

First, in Chapter 10, you will learn about Energy by doing some simple practical experiments. And you will also learn about two important Yogic concepts/practices – "Mudra" (hand positioning) and "Bandha" (internal body locks) – that will help you become familiar with some ways to best utilize Energy during your Pranayama and other practices.

Chapter 11 is your "Pranayama 101" in which you will begin to learn about what I call "active Pranayama." You will learn some very simple, useful Basic Pranayama.

And then in Chapters 12-15 you will learn four Pranayama that can in some sense be considered "area purifiers" – Kapalabhati (the head and chest), Nadi Shodana (the area of the heart), Agni Sara (the belly), and Asvini Mudra (the lower torso).

I have grouped these four together because they can be very potent when practiced together. As such they can provide a fairly complete purification of major aspects of the body's Subtle Energy system. Each of the four can also of course be very profitably practiced by itself or in some other construct with other Pranayama.

Note also that all four of them not only purify you, but actually start you running Energy through your subtle channels. In one sense the sequence "awakens," (my term), the subtle body – "Energy Awakening" – and readies you for deeper Energy work.

Of the four, Kapalabhati (or Kapalabhati's cousin, Bhastrika) and Nadi Shodana are, to my knowledge, the "Big Two" of Pranayama: they are the two most widely-suggested Pranayama practices. Therefore they are, deservedly, examined here in some detail.

And finally, Chapter 16 introduces you to Ujjayi Breathing, a basic and important Pranayama with which you can delve more deeply into what I call the "Energy Rising" aspects of Pranayama.

10

Energy 101

The Basics

This chapter will give you an idea of how you can very much impact the Energy in your body with:

Mudra: Hand-Finger Positions
and
Bandha: Interior-Body Locks

Both can be beneficially utilized during Pranayama and allied practices.

The Basic Truths

You can learn to consciously feel and even "run" Energy in your body, to good effect. There are tools to use to do this.

Different hand/finger positions can be called, in Yogic terminology, "Mudras." They are said to have different effects on your body and its Energies. My personal experience has in fact verified this – I have found that Mudras can have a <u>big</u> effect – and I have therefore incorporated appropriate Mudras into many of my practices.

Even from a Non-Yogic physiological perspective, hands are important. For example: from observing my students lying down in Savasana over the years I have concluded that the degree of their mental/emotional tension is often mirrored in tension in their hands.

The different Locks seal in Energy so that it is directed or kept or forced or channeled into the desired places during your practice, rather than dissipated or allowed to go into the wrong places.

There are three major Interior-Body Locks, (in Yogic terminology "Bandhas"): Root Lock, Belly Lock and Chin Lock. They were previously discussed in the "Definitions" section.

We will revisit both these concepts – Mudra and Bandha – again, later, in discussing various Pranayama.

Finger-Positioning Basics:
Mudras, Chakras & Energy

There are seven possible thumb-tip to-fingertip positions:
Thumb to index fingertip.
Thumb to the notch between the index and middle fingertips.
Thumb to middle fingertip.
Thumb to the notch between the middle and ring fingertips.
Thumb to ring fingertip.
Thumb to the notch between the ring and little fingertips.
Thumb to little fingertip.

There are also seven major Chakras, (Energy Points/Areas in the body), the seven which were mentioned on the "Definitions" page.

Each of the seven thumb-finger positions are, in my considered opinion, related, somehow, to the seven Chakra areas:

Thumb - Index finger	= 7th Chakra	Top of Head
Thumb - Index/Middle finger notch	= 6th Chakra	Third Eye
Thumb - Middle finger	= 5th Chakra	Lower Throat
Thumb - Middle/Ring finger notch	= 4th Chakra	Heart
Thumb - Ring finger	= 3rd Chakra	Solar Plexus
Thumb - Ring/Little finger notch	= 2d Chakra	Abdomen
Thumb - Little finger	= 1st Chakra	Tailbone

Up and Down Energy Demo

If you yourself have not yet experienced the importance of finger/hand position in relation to Energy in the body, I suggest you try out a simple technique that I use in my Yoga classes to demonstrate its relevance to my new students.

Sit with your hands resting on your thighs, palms up. Get yourself at least relatively deeply calmed, (by Pranayama or Meditation if you wish). Then "be" – i.e., put yourself – <u>up in your head</u>, with the tips of both your <u>thumbs</u> against the tips of your <u>index fingers</u>.

Now. Quickly. Transfer the tips of both your thumbs from your index fingers to the tips of your <u>middle fingers</u>.

See if you can feel/sense Energy descend down the body.

Now. Quickly. Take your thumb-tips from your middle fingers to the tips of your <u>ring fingers</u>.

See if you are sensitized to the fact that your Energy now sinks even lower.

Now. Quickly. Take your thumb-tips to the tips of your little fingers.

See if you can feel the Energy sink even lower.

Now. Quickly. Switch both thumbs back from the little fingers to the <u>index fingers</u> once again.

Feel the Energy go zinging back up.

In my experience, when they try this technique for the first time many if not most students get an indication of some sort of Mudra-Energy relationship.

Right-Left Energy Demo

Here's another demonstration of the Mudra-Energy relationship. Sit once again with tips of your thumbs on the tips of your index fingers.

Now, press your right thumb <u>strongly</u> into your right index finger. You may feel an Energy-shift to the right side of your body.

Now: relax that pressure and instead press your left thumb strongly into your left index finger. Feel the Energy sway to the left.

Now: press back and forth, right-left, right-left. Notice the imbalance you create. Feel the Energy rock back and forth in the body.

Now, finally: press equally once again. Feel the balance. And feel how good it is!

Calming versus Jazzing-Up Energy Demo

To feel what even a basic a thumb-finger position can do to your mental/physical/emotional state sit calmly with your hands resting on your thighs and your palms facing upwards or sideways towards each other. Put your hands into the Mudra that has your thumb-tips resting in the notch between the tips of your index and middle fingers, and pushing slightly into your fingertips. This is the calming position.

Now: switch your thumb-tips around to the front of your fingers, so that the fingernails of your two fingers are now pressing into the back of your thumb tips. This is the energizing/jazzing up position. Notice how you feel. Notice the Energetic difference.

If you don't feel the difference right away go back and forth between the two positions.

Thumb-Tapping Energy Flow Demo

Here's another finger-positioning exercise that might bring you a deeper understanding of the Mudra-Chakra relationship, and also of Energy movement.

Tap your thumbs lightly on your fingertips, over and over, at each of the seven thumb-to-finger positions previously listed. Tap for a while on one, then go to another and tap it, etc. This may bring you a sense of the Energy Center that is somehow connected to that particular position.

Or you may of course just try holding your thumbs in the various positions without tapping.

A Mudra-Chakra Example

The Mudra-Chakra associations that I have listed at the start of this chapter came to me through my personal practice. Only after having experienced them did I find from my research that other practitioners had reached the same conclusions.

I'll give you just one example. The physically-experienced association I feel between the Heart (4th) Chakra and the Mudra of having the thumb-tips in the notch between the tips of the middle and ring fingers has been recognized in India and formalized in what is called the Heart Mudra, ("Hridaya Mudra").

In some versions of Hridaya Mudra, along with your thumb-tips being held between the tips of your middle and ring fingers, the nail of your index finger is pressed against the base of your thumb, and your little finger is held out straight. However I myself do not practice or teach it that way.

So. This is more advanced Energy work. But if you want to try it, sit, palms up, hands resting on thighs. Take the Mudra. See if you somehow feel some sort of a difference.

If not, stay seated a while with the fingers of both hands in the Mudra and see if you can eventually locate/experience a different feeling in the area of the heart. (Or even a happiness in the upper arms, i.e, near the level of the heart).

Or: try raising your arms up, to bring your hands and the Mudra closer to your heart. Sit there and experience.

Body-Mind-Spirit Connectivity

As you might suspect from the above discussion, certain finger positions, if held during individual Pranayama, enhance the Pranayama. We will discuss later in this volume how you can utilize these associations during some of the Pranayama. And in later volumes we will discuss how they can be utilized in other, related practices.

So. If you are able to experience all these internal Energy changes just by making minor adjustments with your <u>fingers,</u> does this mean that if you tweak one aspect of your posture, or area of your body, it will affect the Energy in your entire being?

Ah. Welcome to Yoga.

Hands/Fingers Energy Flow Demo

Here are two further demos which can bring home to you the fact that you can "run" Energy in your body. In both we will use hand and arm positioning.

Our body is by design forward-facing, and thus frontward-biased, but if our postures and Energies are excessively forward-thrusting, we tend to be too jazzed up.

And, if that is the case it is better – in order to become more calm and "grounded" and thus be able to utilize our Energy in a more effective manner – to rein in our forward-thrusting Energy. To take it, (to "Run it"), <u>backwards</u>.

Let's demonstrate this in ways you can easily test.

You can try the first demo when you are driving a car, perhaps on a freeway, and are over-hurried, or ensnared in slow traffic, and maybe even anxious, or angry, or at least filled with impatience. Take your right hand off the wheel (if you are right-handed) and rest it in your lap, with your fingers curled back towards your torso. Then adjust your left hand on the wheel so that its fingers are also pointing more backwards, towards your body.

You should calm down <u>immediately</u>.

The forward flow of your Energy has been abated. It may even become difficult to force yourself to drive fast. You have managed – or "run" – your Energy Flow. And you have done this just with a very simple and minor external postural adjustment. Just the fingers and the hands.

The second demo is similar. Again you can try it while driving. Position your hands high on the steering wheel with your palms facing forward. Then drop your hands down and hold on to the bottom portion of the wheel with your hands rotated so that your palms are now facing you. You should feel more aggressive in the upper position, more calm in the lower.

Energy & Internal Posture

You can also manage your Energy by consciously-assumed <u>internal</u>-body configurations, without changing your external posture. I'll give you another demo to play with, and then will discuss some Bandhas.

Energy Flow Demo: "Eye Energy"

Once again in a traffic jam, or some such situation when you are similarly ensnarled or agitated, you can test "running" Energy with <u>internal</u> body activity. Try to consciously take the Energy from the <u>outer</u> <u>corners</u> of your eyes backwards, either through your head, or along your temples, back towards the rear of your head.

Don't take back the eyes themselves, physically, but just the Energy there.

You should experience the same instant calming effect that you did when you changed your hand positions in the car in our earlier demo.

And now – if you wish to go further – first take this Energy back to the back of the head, and <u>then</u>, from there, down your back, (this may happen by itself). If you do this you will relax even more. Your tense, hunched-up shoulders will relax of their own accord.

I utilize this "Eye Energy" principle in my Yoga classes when I bring my students out of Corpse Pose, ("Savasana"). I often tell them to open their eyes as they are lying there, but to try to keep their eyes soft, (rather than being "hard-eyed" and reaching out and grabbing with those hard eyes), and to be receptive through the outer corners of their eyes.

Being soft-eyed helps them to retain the calm of the Savasana even though they are now lying there with their eyes open.

Note: if you doubt the truth of "hard eyes" versus "soft eyes," notice what happens to your eyes the next time you see someone who greatly attracts you, sexually.

Bandhas: Interior-Body Locks

We will now define, and discuss my opinions about, the three major "Locks" in Yoga: Root Lock, Belly Lock and Chin Lock. Please realize that, as with many things in Yoga, there are significantly differing opinions about even the basics of these entities.

Root Lock: "Mula Bandha"

Mula Bandha is perhaps the primary Lock in Yoga. It is considered so important that entire books have been written about it. With of course, as stated above, differing opinions.

I feel there are various ways, progressively more subtle, that you yourself might want to consider trying in order to establish Mula Bandha:

(1) As a beginner, don't over-think it. Don't feel clueless and inadequate. Just clench your butt or, more particularly, clench your anal sphincter, as if you have to prevent yourself from defecating. The anal sphincter thus feels like it moves slightly up into the body. Hold it there. This, in itself, is in fact, according to some Yogic schools of thought, Mula Bandha.

(2) An intermediate stage might involve learning to lift the area between your anus and your genitals, that is, your perineum. You might practice by clenching the anal sphincter, and the urethral sphincter, together and individually; learning to discriminate between the two; and then trying to lift the perineum between them without overly clenching either of the sphincters themselves.

(3) Later, (perhaps), learn to lift the pelvic floor by doing the lifting internally, higher up. There are at least three ways of thinking about this.

A. Learn to establish a clenching deep up inside the anus, not at the anal aperture but about "four finger-widths" up inside.
B. Or – women can think: lift the area of the cervix. Or can think: lift the ovaries. Or: do a Kegel.
C. Or – men can think: lift the internal area where the head of the penis would be, if the penis was erect but inverted diagonally up into the body, mimicking its placement near the cervix in intercourse. Once found, this area is, at least to me, easily accessed and lifted.

<u>An "Ashtanga Yoga" Alternative</u>. I like the way of <u>accessing</u> Mula Bandha as described by Tim Miller, a senior teacher from the "Ashtanga Yoga" school of thought (re-)founded by Pattabhi Jois. Seated, begin an Inhale from the root of your tailbone. And as you begin, pull your breath forward from your tailbone towards your pubic bone. Also begin to stretch up your lower abdomen. Pausing, you can become aware of what Ashtanga Yoga believes to be Mula Bandha engaging. (Yoga Journal, May/June 2003, page 40).

This engagement is in the same area as described in options B and C above. I like the grounded feeling this route, (pun intended), supplies.

Another correct way to think of Mula Bandha, however, may be more subtle. In that regard, the words of other Yoga Teachers once again precisely echo my feelings:

> "I look at Root Bond more as an energetic response to a whole chain of peripheral movements and actions…"
>
> > Yoga Teacher Richard Rosen
> > <u>Pranayama Beyond the Fundamentals</u>
> > p 96

> "Where we'd like to end up with mulabandha/asvini is with spontaneous subtle movements as ecstatic energy moves naturally inside us."
>
> > Yoga Teacher "Yogani"
> > <u>Advanced Yoga Practices</u>, p 193

These both correspond to my experience: not only am I able to consciously induce Mula Bandha by the above-described internal lifting, but it can also spontaneously occur as a reaction to activity in the lower abdomen.

If you yourself feel physically light and upflowing, and/or your mood instantly perks up (if only subtly), then you've got it.

If your Energy sensitivity is well-developed you may feel Mula Bandha send Energy right up the body and into the head. You want this.

Why do you want this? That question goes to the important, related question:

Why do you want to do Mula Bandha?

To bring Energy up.

What Energy?

Ah. There are at least two ways of looking at it.

The first is that you wish to bring <u>sexual</u> energy up.

The second is that you wish to bring "<u>Kundalini</u>" Energy up.

So. One way to look at the bringing up of sexual energy is that (1) in a male this energy, (semen), is manufactured in the testes, so that the activation of a "First Chakra" located at the male perineum would be close to it and thus effective; while (2) in a female the energy, (ova), is manufactured in the ovaries, which are close in the horizontal plane to the cervix, which is the area the woman is therefore often advised to activate.

As for "Kundalini" Energy. One theory – to which I currently subscribe – is that it resides close to the base of the tailbone, (coccyx). And this base, or tip, of the coccyx is located behind and above the anal canal, (the channel which the anal sphincters grip). Thus the clenching of the anal sphincters is more likely to activate that area than would lifting the perineum.

ENERGY 101

But better: if you locate/bring your lifting up a bit further up in the body, (Options B and C above), you bring the lifting right to the area near the tip of the tailbone.

The cervix in women, and in men the tip of an inverted penis – (that mimics the placement of the cervix) – both locate you with more precision in front of the tip of the tailbone.

Bingo.

Well. It's theory, isn't it?

So, in any event, _why_ do we want to bring Energy up?

One (true) answer is that when you've done it you won't have to ask.

A perhaps more elucidating answer – if you subscribe, as I currently do, to the Kundalini theory – is that for some reason, (perhaps because the Kundalini area is a concentrated repository of Universal Energy, or "Prana," or what I am in this Guidebook calling "Energy"), bringing this "Kundalini" Energy up through your subtle body channels and Chakras purifies them, and you – with resultant physical and spiritual benefits.

Asana Note: Mula Bandha and Uddiyana Bandha are also very helpful, indeed important, safety tools, to be engaged during many Yogic poses.

Belly Lock: "Uddiyana Bandha"

The version I currently subscribe to: with a forceful _Exhale_ you take the area of your solar plexus, (just below your rib cage), both _in_ and _up_. Uddiyana Bandha refers to "flying upward." This in essence refers, I believe, to the fact that this lock, like Mula Bandha, is helpful in moving Energy up the body.

Uddiyana Bandha tugs or draws or sends or induces Energy up the body.

Calling this Lock a "Belly Lock" or an "Abdominal Lock" is – in my opinion – yet another example of the commonplace event of an oversimplification that has somehow stuck. For – again, this is my opinion – what is being clenched inward is not the belly, not all the abdominal musculature, but more specifically an area higher up, around the solar plexus.

Opinions, however, differ – as, sigh, always – as to just what and where to clench, and how.

When to Apply Uddiyana

Opinions can also differ about whether – when you are applying Uddiyana Bandha in order to enhance upward Energy flow – it is meant to be applied during or at the end of an Exhale, or during or at the end of an Inhale.

I personally like it during an Exhale, a Suspension (after an Exhale), or a Retention (after an Inhale). Not during an Inhale. I find it difficult to draw my upper belly both in and up <u>during</u> an Inhale.

Uddiyana Bandha can be induced by Mula Bandha. I myself like establishing Belly Lock in conjunction with Root Lock.

Also, Uddiyana Bandha might itself induce Chin Lock (Jalandhara Bandha) – the chin may seem to be tugged downward.

Uddiyana Bandha Alternatives

Uddiyana Bandha is taught in other ways:

Some schools of thought place the lockage lower down the torso.

I posit, however, that Root Lock is designed to act upon the First and Second Chakra areas in the lower abdominal area, and that thus Belly Lock can rightfully be expected to act upon the Third Chakra area, at the solar plexus. And I myself feel it most vigorously there.

It is also sometimes taught as a "false inhale," (a rib cage expansion), after a forceful <u>Exhale</u>, or even without having forcefully Exhaled. This method purports to draw/tuck Energy further up under the rib cage.

I very much <u>like</u> this version, especially as a stand-alone, as it is useful to demonstrate how establishment of Belly Lock draws Energy up and also how it leads into establishment of Chin Lock. (Again, all three major locks can work together).

So. Experiment. Find what works for you. And in any event: try to have people explain <u>why</u> they propose a certain method.

Chin Lock: "Jalandhara Bandha"

In Jalandhara Bandha you take your chin down into your neck notch and bring your chest up to meet it.

This Lock can be used either to keep Energy up above the throat or down in the torso. Uddiyana Bandha and Ujjayi Breathing are both effective precursors to its establishment.

"Jal" can mean a "net," and "net" implies that this name refers to catching Energy, as it falls down from the head, and preventing it from flowing downward. "Dhara" can mean "stop." Chin Lock can thus be thought of as a net that stops Energy.

There is in fact Yogic theory that states, which I have experienced, that there is an ambrosia-like substance created up in the head, ("amrita"). The theory is that this amrita drips downward, down into the throat, but that it is a good idea to prevent this and keep it upstairs. Under this interpretation, the name Jalandhara makes perfect sense. It is a net to stop the amrita from dripping down.

As will be mentioned later, in various contexts, if you perform a Chin Lock after an Inhale it can be helpful to swallow after you Inhale and right before you apply the Chin Lock.

The Locks are Related

Again:

Root Lock induces/leads naturally into Belly Lock, and even into Chin Lock.

Belly Lock helps induce Root Lock, and leads naturally into/induces Chin Lock; it seems to bring the chin down.

All three are established and held in the Yoga pose called Maha Mudra.

All three work both to fine down the breath and to help run Energy.

11
Pranayama 101

Overview

There are countless Pranayama variations. In this chapter we discuss some very basic ones – Antara Kumbhaka, Dirga Puraka and Dirga Rechaka – which you can use to get a feel for what a practice is like, and which you can continue to use, beneficially, for as long as you wish.

Before you practice, however, on any given day, you might want to determine the relative abilities of your nostrils, in order to assess your capabilities. So we start with Nostril Testing.

Nostril Testing

Technique

It's simple. All you need to do is take a breath in and out of one nostril, with the opposite thumb closing down the other nostril. And then do the same thing with the other nostril.

Why Test?

There are two very good reasons for doing nostril testing at the start of your session:

<u>In order to determine what an appropriate practice might be that day.</u>

It is a very good idea to know what to expect from your body in any given session, so that you don't push yourself too far and/or don't feel disappointed because things don't seem to be going as "well" as in other sessions.

And the condition of each nostril can tell you what to expect. Nostril testing, if done over time, sensitizes you: you realize with some certainty how open you are on any particular day, and thus know whether you might need to adjust your Pranayama practice accordingly

In Pranayama as in Asana you should take what is available, what is given to you on any particular day, with the knowledge that it is entirely normal for your capabilities to vary tremendously. Pranayama is <u>not</u> a competition with yourself, with ever-expansive targets-to-be-met.

<u>In order to determine your strong and weak nostrils.</u>

When you test your nostrils you note the relative degree of difficulty in Inhaling and Exhaling on each side. This indicates their relative "strength," and this knowledge gives you the option of starting your Nadi Shodana with your weaker nostril or your stronger one. (The reasoning behind starting one way or the other will be explained in the chapter on Nadi Shodana.)

Nostril Condition Options

There are three blockage possibilities. Right nostril more blocked. Left nostril more blocked. Both nostrils relatively similarly restricted or open.

Expect good results in Pranayama when both nostrils are open. (Some Yogic literature posits that Dawn and Dusk and Noon and Midnight are the times when this is likely to beneficially occur.)

Caveat: over time I have found that I personally get my best result when my left nostril is just slightly blocked, and when my right is a little more blocked than the left. If my nostrils are completely open I don't usually get as good results. It's just too easy to Inhale, and so my Inhale may not achieve a desirable length.

Nostril Blockage Curing

If there is a blockage in a nostril, or a big imbalance between the nostrils, then you have some curative options to try to open and balance your nostrils a bit:

(1) Do some more Single-Nostril Breathing. Just continue to breathe in and out of one nostril, as you did in your test. Take four or five breaths in and out through your more-closed nostril, keeping the other nostril closed with a finger or thumb.

And then, to maintain balance, do four or five more through the more-open nostril.

Repeat if you want.

(2) Or you might in the alternative, (or also), try lying on your side with the blocked nostril higher than the open nostril, so things have a chance to drain.

Note that in a "blocked" situation you are *not* trying to completely open up the nostrils. You are just trying to even out the playing field a bit. You are once again seeking balance and symmetry.

(3) If there is a complete imbalance/blockage, (as when you have a cold), do not necessarily expect to do Pranayama. You might give it up for that day, and just do Meditation or Asana. Or try "Therapeutic Kapalabhati" as discussed in the Kapalabhati chapter that follows this chapter.

But: if you regularly start your day with a Hot Shower and/or use a Neti Pot, (Neti Pot use will be discussed in Volume II), you should expect to be open enough – more so if you do Asana, (especially Inversions), and Pranayama regularly – to practice nearly every day of the year.

Because, if you embrace the package listed in the above paragraph, you should find, over time, that you are not as susceptible to severe colds, debilitating runny noses, etc.

Basic Pranayama

When you are starting out in Pranayama you might if you wish practice these basic Pranayama:

1. Holding your Breath after an Inhale - "Antara Kumbhaka"
2. Making your Inhale long - "Dirga Puraka"
3. Making your Exhale long - "Dirga Rechaka"

These are beginners' practices that will enhance your ability to practice the more complex Pranayama that follow in this Guidebook. And in this guise they are essentially training vehicles. But all three of them can also be, in their more advanced forms, very potent indeed, and will be discussed in that context in Volume II.

Holding Your Breath after an Inhale (Antara Kumbhaka)

This Pranayama technique is simply holding your breath after an Inhale. And – because in it you do not ordinarily deprive yourself of oxygen to the extent that you might do in Bahya Kumbhaka, (holding your breath after an Exhale) – it might therefore be considered more safe. When of course practiced with prudence.

Inhale Big, Into the Chest

Start with a normal Exhale. Then Inhale up your torso. But don't let the breath come up into the throat and create too much pressure. Take it to the back of the upper torso. Keep the air wide at the level of the heart. Puff/expand your chest out.

Establish a Chin Lock, or All Three Locks

Initially it may be easier for you to concentrate, as you are holding your breath, by establishing and holding just a Chin Lock. With time though, as you become more proficient, it may be helpful to establish and hold a full Root Lock as well as a <u>Mini</u> Belly Lock.

A Mini Belly Lock is basically a subtle pulling in and up at the Solar Plexus. A full Belly Lock is not appropriate during a Retention after an Inhale.

Count

Now, as you are holding your breath, count, in order to establish where your Edge is. Again: your Edge is how long you can hold your breath without any debilitating discomfort.

I count by 20's or 30's in this Pranayama, (counting 1 to 20 or 30 and repeating), because larger numbers seem too complex for my brain to take in, and because I have found that when I count by 20's or 30's I can also hold my breath longer.

If you do this I suggest you transfer your thumb-tip to a different fingertip after each 20/30-count, to keep track of where you are.

Hold Your Breath for As Long As You Prudently Can

Become soft inside the confines of the pose. You may concentrate your mind on the repetition of the numbers of your count. Or you might want to focus your mind between your shoulder blades, or on the back of your head or neck, or on the air just outside your chest. Or wherever calms you best, in order to keep your mind quiescent.

The keys here are to keep your mind soft and to keep your mid and lower torso internally soft. Quiet mind, quiet body.

Notice if you feel wide at the collarbones.

The duration in which you can remain in Antara Kumbhaka may very well be extended by a voluntary forward and backward head-bobbing. I suggest you make the bobbing minimal and fairly quick. I often do mine somewhat in time with my count.

Build your capacity up to 108, or 120, or 200, or whatever. Counting lets you monitor your progress, but beware of letting the quest for a higher count take over. Again, you are not trying to establish new "personal bests" here, or in any of the Pranayama.

You are not "at bat" when you do Pranayama. You don't have to try to hit home runs.

What you are trying to do here is to go as far as you comfortably can, without a big air-blast or gasping when you finally come out. A big gasp after a long Retention or Suspension can be dangerous.

Exhale and Recover

Exhale. Try to let the air come out slowly and controlled. As you Exhale let your head rise up, out from your Chin Lock..

You may lean back mentally in your Third Eye Area as you sit there recovering. Take at least five normal breaths, many more if necessary. Notice how sweet the breath is. Silently repeat a simple one or two-syllable Mantra for a while if you want. Again, I do not suggest using a complicated Mantra at this point.

Even brief or slight (1) nausea, (2) dizziness or (3) a feeling of panic means that you've gone too far. Use this curative if needed: as you Inhale, press down strongly into your thighs with the back of your wrists; then do an Exhale with a nose-mouth-nose sequence. Doing this sequence <u>two times</u> should release any accumulated pressure.

Note: the initial beneficial effects of Antara Kumbhaka are not felt during the holding itself, but afterwards in this Recovery period. You might, for example, feel as though you are breathing up and down a Central Channel in your body.

> <u>Note Well</u>: the practice of Inhaling and holding your breath is also known as a Pranayama called Murcha (or Murchha), which I believe is Sanskrit for "fainting." And indeed in Murcha you are sometimes taught to go to the extreme of holding your breath until you feel like you are going to faint. I feel this is dangerous and inadvisable. I don't like the concept and I don't use the name.

Extending Your Inhale (Dirga Puraka)
Extending Your Exhale (Dirga Rechaka)

Dirga ("Long") Puraka ("Inhale") is simply a deep nasal Exhale followed by a nasal Inhale that you make as long and slow and subtle as you can possibly make it. You can count as you Inhale, in order to establish your capability.

Dirga ("Long") Rechaka ("Exhale") is, on the other hand, simply a deep nasal Inhale followed by a nasal Exhale that you make as long and slow and subtle as you can possibly make it. Again, you count as you Exhale, to establish your capability.

You may do advanced versions of either Dirga Puraka or Dirga Rechaka by dividing your long and slow and subtle Inhale or Exhale into portions (as many as you wish) with quick soft pauses, (hesitations), between the portions.

Dirga Puraka and Dirga Rechaka are basic practices. They are among those Pranayama that the extraordinarily-experienced Yoga Teacher B.K.S. Iyengar teaches to beginners. They build up respiratory capacity safely.

They can therefore be used initially as training vehicles, to develop your capacity to do the more difficult, (yet, if practiced with caution, also safe), Pranayama in this Guidebook. And, as mentioned above, deeper versions of Dirga Puraka and Dirga Rechaka can be potent advanced techniques, and as such are discussed in Volume II.

My students, however, once introduced to the other Pranayama in this Guidebook, tend to be more inclined to practice them than to do these elementary Pranayama during the Pranayama phase at the end of my Yoga classes.

12

Kapalabhati

The Basic Truths Behind It

Kapalabhati, (kah-pahl-ah-bah-tee), purifies areas of your <u>head</u> – ("kapal" means "head" or "skull") – and your <u>upper torso</u>. It also prepares those areas to receive the Energy you will if you wish bring up from your lower body with your later Pranayama.

Kapalabhati clears pathways. In and of itself, it can calm you down. It can also be a very nice vehicle for putting yourself into your Third Eye Area.

Kapalabhati can teach you how the Mind, Breath and Body can come together as one.

<u>Kapalabhati is not appropriate for those with unmedicated high blood pressure.</u>
<u>Kapalabhati is not appropriate for pregnant women.</u>

The Basics

In Kapalabhati, (sometimes spelled Kapalbhati), you create a forceful Exhalation <u>out</u> through the nose by strongly jerking in your <u>solar plexus</u>, (in the notch just below the center of your rib cage).

Or, better, if you can, by jerking in and <u>up</u>.

You then let your Inhale occur naturally. Then you jerk again. You do this over and over, at speed, counting your breaths as you do.

There are several levels of Kapalabhati. Initially you might want to aim to achieve 108 Inhales/Exhales in a minute.

Later, (much, much later), you might want to develop an ability to do thousands, consecutively, over a much longer period of time. This much higher level of practice will be discussed in Volumes II and III.

Kapalabhati Works Best "Up-Front"

Experience has convinced me that it is best to practice Kapalabhati at or very near the start of the active Pranayama portion of your practice session.

This is because Kapalabhati – although a potent Pranayama in itself – also very much enhances your ability to do the Pranayama that follow it. It <u>bounces</u> you into your active Pranayama phase, prepares your Energy systems, opens up your head and chest and respiratory system, calms you down, and sets you up for further Pranayama.

Because Kapalabhati is forceful it heats and clears your respiratory system. You become warm and open for your following Pranayama, instead of cold and crimped. Kapalabhati also oxygenates you, which helps you to better perform any oxygen-depleting Pranayama that follow. My Nadi Shodana, (if it is, as it is often, my next Pranayama), is never as effective if I do it without having done some Kapalabhati first.

That said, it's a balancing act. If you don't do Kapalabhati first, the Pranayama that follow may not be as effective. But if your Kapalabhati is so strenuous that it stresses your respiratory system, it can greatly degrade your ability to perform, at the very least, your next Pranayama.

Kapalabhati is one of the two Pranayama best suited to be your first active Pranayama. I consider "Single-Nostril Breathing," which will be discussed in Volume II, to be the other good "starter Pranayama" for the "active" portion of your session. (It can be a good starter substitute for Kapalabhati for those with unmedicated high blood pressure.)

Chapter Overview

The rest of this chapter is divided into four sections:

1. Techniques of Basic Kapalabhati
2. Affected Areas
3. Post-Kapalabhati
4. Other Aspects of Kapalabhati

Techniques of Basic Kapalabhati

Remember that you should be sitting erect, that is, sitting straight up with your spine in its natural curves. Any slouch, however slight, degrades the practice. You may wish to roll your shoulders slightly back and take your shoulder blades slightly down to prevent slouching.

And again, your initial practice might be to learn to do Kapalabhati over and over for one minute, aiming to reach 108 breaths. If you can reach 108 Inhale/Exhales in under one minute, you can stop.

If and when you can do 108 easily – with no stress, and with the same force and speed throughout – you can try for 120 breaths in one minute. Most of the sources I have studied are in concert: no more than 120. And I agree that that is a very good speed for a beginner to stick with. (But see later.)

Why a 120 maximum? Why 108?

120 breaths per minute seems to me, from experience, a good, viable, safe maximum rate for Kapalabhati, at least for beginners. Anything more than that may sacrifice quality.

Don't let it bother you if you can't reach 108 or 120 when you start up your practice. Over the months and years you should be able to achieve them both. And, with time, 120 should become easier to reach, more unforced, with your last 30 breaths becoming as easy as your first 30.

Why 108? The number has a plethora of "mystical" or religious meanings, not only in Hinduism, but also in Islam and Buddhism. And it has been endowed with all sorts of meanings and explanations – including numerological and astrological ones – of its "power." (Interesting irrelevant fact: in some areas of India 108 is used as the equivalent of the 911 emergency telephone number used in America.)

It seems to me possible that the Indian religious/mystical 108 was grafted onto/incorporated into Pranayama in order to give an Indian practitioner an easily recognizable, achievable goal.

On a practical plane, however, avoidance of a building-up of pressure in the ears during Kapalabhati may be why a 120-count maximum has been emphasized. It may well be that 120 is considered to be the upper end of a safe zone of repetitions.

Some Yogic schools of thought teach a lesser maximum number. As always, strive to find what is effective for you.

All that said, my experience has shown me that you can safely go to a 150-count per minute, once you have become capable of doing this sort of advanced practice. I tried this for the first time after a few of my more advanced students told me they were not getting their best results stopping at 120, but by going on to 150. I tried it. It worked well for me. I adopted it in my personal practice.

And then, over time, it even became easy for me to do 180-breaths which is my current personal practice speed for a one-minute practice. I am _not_ advocating this for beginners.

Getting Into It

The way I myself begin – which works very well for me – is with a single deep sharp Exhale. This seems to nicely jump-start the jerking Exhales. After that Exhale, and after a slight pause, I can get right into the rhythm of the jerking.

Alternatively you can try doing a few test jerk-Exhales before you actually commence your round, just to get your system into the swing of things. This is especially helpful when your throat is tight or you have an excess of saliva.

Another reason that you might want to do a couple of forceful test-Exhales is to see if there is snot in your nose which will be spewed out by the Exhale. (Maybe have tissues handy?) Best, yes, to get this out of the way before you get into your actual Kapalabhati.

If you do have trouble getting into the swing of things, I also suggest that you might want to try starting slowly at the beginning of your Kapalabhati, and then build momentum, (like a train chug-chug-chugging out of the station). That way you will not stress your nostrils right off the bat.

Your Chin, Mouth and Tongue

Kapalabhati can work with your chin either slightly raised, held at a normal level or dropped slightly down. Experiment. See which position opens or loosens the "knot" or "blockage" at your throat, and allows your Breath and Energy to come up from your solar plexus more easily. (Dropping your chin down seems to help in focusing your attention on your Third Eye. However I am fond of chin up.)

If you keep your lips or teeth just slightly open as you do Kapalabhati, it may help counter any build-up of pressure in the ears. But don't mouth-breathe.

Or, you may want to practice with your mouth shut, which can be especially helpful if you are doing an extended practice, as it helps counter the tendency of the mouth to become dry.

Your Hands and Feet

Rolling your <u>hands</u> slightly open externally as they rest on your thighs may help open you to Kapalabhati. On the other hand, I find that rolling the <u>wrists</u> inwards towards each other helps to stabilize the body and to enable a lengthy Kapalabhati session.

I suggest that the fingers of each of your hands be cupped firmly together, with your hands in the Third Eye Mudra position, i.e., with your thumb-tips resting in the notch between the tips of your index and middle fingers. Firmly together is best. Not tightly together, not loosely, but moderately.

It is helpful to press your feet – more particularly the front of your foot, including your toes – lightly but firmly into the floor:

> (1) Pushing the balls of the feet into the floor both straightens the body and helps Energy to rise.

> (2) Again, this is especially helpful when you are doing a lengthy Kapalabhati. And when things get tough, try pressing a bit harder with the inner edges of the front of the foot, the big toe and second toe area.

The "positional totality" of the balls of your feet pressing into the floor, your wrists cocked towards each other, and your fingers cupped together all meshes together to provide a very useful stability.

Are You Kapalabhati-Challenged?

Some people can get into the "Jerking-In Exhale/Normal Inhale" rhythm very easily. For other people it's a bit of a challenge. They can't for the life of them get into the flow of it. They keep Inhaling as they jerk in. It's as maddeningly difficult for them as if they are trying to pat the top of their head and rub their bellies at the same time.

If this is in fact the case for you, don't despair: the good news is that, either rather quickly or over what seems like an agonizingly long time, Kapalabhati <u>can</u> be learned.

What I have these challenged students do is put their index finger into their belly-button. Then have them push their finger in, strongly, and at the same time Exhale. They do this very slowly to begin with, just trying to get the muscle memory. And then eventually they speed up. Finger-push/Exhale. Finger-push/Exhale. And finally, when they feel able, they get rid of their "training finger" and fly solo.

Note: I also often tell beginning students to jerk their belly-buttons in, (an easier action than jerking the solar plexus), just to get them into the swing of things. But in my opinion you should learn eventually to do the jerking totally in the area of the solar plexus, not lower.

Speed, Depth & Force

In Kapalabhati you can jerk in and release out at a low speed or at a high speed; with a deep jerking or a shallow jerking.

In fact, during a round, your body may well automatically slow you down or speed you up as you go along, and/or make you go deep or shallow. Sometimes the body will take you spontaneously into a series of extremely fast breaths – like a "Kapalabhati windsprint" – and then settle back down into your slower speed. (Sometimes however it may just keep accelerating and accelerating until you finally put your foot down and stop it from happening.)

Do what feels good.

I do suggest that <u>initially</u> you might want to work towards being able to practice as forcefully and deeply and quickly as you can <u>without stress</u>. I suggest this because I think it builds up the power of your muscles, and your respiratory capacity. And with time you can go longer and longer, which brings more potent results. And of course increased respiratory ability will be very helpful in your other Pranayama, as well as in your life.

With time and experience, however, you might want to go more subtly, slowly and deeply into an emphasis on the Energy-movement aspects of the practice.

You may well notice, over the years, that your regular practice of Kapalabhati has enhanced your voice as well as your breathing capabilities. It seems similar in some small sense, I hazard, to operatic training.

Jerk In and UP

Kapalabhati basically takes your solar plexus area, at speed, in and out of the Yogic Lock called Uddiyana Bandha – rather than applying and holding the Lock. If you can learn to go not just in but in <u>and</u> <u>UP</u> it can be even more potent. You are using the Kapalabhati to force Energy up towards your Third Eye Area. You may even sense it bouncing up against your inner skull.

Again, remember that you are using the <u>solar plexus</u> area to jerk in and up; you are not utilizing the lower abdomen; the belly does not roll way out and then get jerked back in. The area of physical activity commences at the solar plexus and involves the chest under the ribs. It should be confined to those areas.

Keep the solar plexus area of the belly fluid and flexible as it does the work. The rest of the torso should remain relatively placid, or, even better, still. And your head should not be jerking around like a fish flopping around on the ground.

Mental Focus Options

You may find it helpful, after you have started, to try to keep yourself lightly focused in your Third Eye Area (the Sixth Chakra). This may help you in sensing Energy coming up to that area.

Another beneficial outcome of this Third Eye Area focus is that it helps keep your body straight. Remember however that, although your spine is kept erect, it is helpful in this regard to keep your chin slightly tilted down.

You may find it particularly helpful to try to hold fast to an image of the face of a loved one in your Third Eye Area. I myself have found that this tremendously empowers the breathing.

Or you may keep your mind focused on the area of the solar plexus, (the Third Chakra).

Or you may if you wish go back and forth with your focus between your Third Eye Area and your solar plexus – or your Third Eye Area, solar plexus and <u>throat</u>.

Or, as you count to 108, or 120, focus your mind on your counting.

In any event, try not to think. Thinking detracts from the potency of Pranayama.

The Counting is Tough

The mind seems to have a difficult time wrapping itself around large numbers when breathing at speed. To counter this I suggest that you might want to count by 20's or 30's or 50's rather than counting from 1 to 108, or from 1 to 120.

From long practice I myself can count easily by 30's now and not lose track of where I am at overall – if I am doing a short Kapalabhati. However, until you develop that ability what you might do is to count from 1 to 30 with the tips of your left thumb and left index finger together (as your hands rest on your thighs.) Then count from 1 to 30 again, but this time with your thumb tip against the tip of your middle finger. For 60-90 go to the tip of your ring finger. And then finally, for 90-120, go to the tip of your little finger.

This should get you to 120 without any big-number brain-fuzziness. The position of your thumb assists you in remembering where you are in your count.

When you develop the ability to go past 120 your other hand can also come into play: you transfer your thumb-tip from fingertip to fingertip, signaling you when each 120-count has been performed. This is important. Without this concrete, physical aid the mind can lose count.

Kapalabhati Do's & Don'ts

If you feel any pressure building up in the ears, make sure your mouth is at least slightly open and leave it open. If the pressure doesn't go away as you continue to perform Kapalabhati with your mouth open:

<u>Stop! You are trying too hard!</u>

Don't distress your nostrils! (Note that, especially if you are practicing fast and vigorously and doing a lengthy Kapalabhati, your nostrils may even start to <u>burn</u>. Stop!)

Don't distress your respiratory system!

If your throat starts to dry up, Stop! You do not want a dry, raspy throat in the later Pranayama.

Don't snork! If you are snorking you are trying too hard.

Do keep your shoulders relaxed.

Do not clench your toes. Unclench your toes!

Don't lean sideways. Be equal and heavy into the sitz-bones. You want to feel equal on both sides of your torso. This is one reason to sit with your feet square into the floor rather than putting the soles of your feet together.

Don't worry if Kapalabhati (or any other Pranayama) induces burping, yawning or swallowing. Who – even in a room full of other Yoga students – cares?

Affected Areas

I believe that Kapalabhati is aimed at, and works in, the area of the head and upper torso, down to and including the solar plexus. It opens up the chest for breathing. It energizes the upper body. It opens the head marvelously. It takes you up and out of emotion.

Many, if not most, of us have a fairly powerful Energetic block in the throat area that we must deal with in order to allow Energy to flow properly through the body. Kapalabhati, especially in its advanced modes, (discussed in Volume II) can serve to "scour" the throat area, unlocking it Energetically.

The focus in Kapalabhati is therefore on the upper body. Rightfully so, in my estimation, for an initial Pranayama, because our gross breathing apparatus is located up there.

And, putting this focus into a Chakra context, I experience Kapalabhati as opening/working/clarifying/purifying the Solar Plexus, Throat and Third Eye Chakras, encompassing the upper torso and head.

KAPALABHATI

Note that it does not seem, to me, to especially work the Heart Chakra. However, Nadi Shodana, the next Pranayama in the "Series of Four" Pranayama, takes care of that lack.

I have asked myself why Kapalabhati does not seem to affect the Heart Chakra area for me and why Nadi Shodana does. And the answer is, I don't know.

Further evidence regarding this upper body focus: as discussed below, during Kapalabhati I sometimes run Energy lines from my head down <u>to</u> my solar plexus. It does not, however, feel right to run these lines any <u>lower</u> than the solar plexus, nor have I been able to successfully do so.

I cannot completely explain why Kapalabhati seems to focus its effects on this upper body area. But I was gratified to discover the following:

> "One old guide claims that it [Kapalabhati] stimulates the energy centers at the solar plexus (manipura-Chakra) and the so-called Third Eye, or ajna-Chakra, at the middle of the forehead."
>
> Yoga Teacher Richard Rosen
> <u>The Yoga of Breath</u>, p 230

Ah-ha! Yes. Just so. Good. I so claim, now, too.

Sidetrack: Richard Rosen

> Over the years I have studied both contemporary and ancient sources on Pranayama. Most of them seem to merely hint at things or to set out bare-bones instruction.
>
> I believe these inadequacies exist, in part, because (1) words are not entirely suitable to describe what is happening to us; (2) many writers resort therefore to poesy and analogy; (3) many Yogic practices have been deemed, rightfully or wrongfully, inappropriate for everyone, and therefore have been cloaked, leaving much to instruction from an individual's "guru" who

can assess a student's suitability to receive them; and (4) Yoga was passed down primarily orally, so written works tended to be less treatises than easily memorized lecture notes, designed to prompt the "gurus."

Thus most of this book consists of things which have come to me during my own practice. I almost therefore entitled the book <u>Pranayama Self-Taught</u> as, in one sense, a play on words regarding received knowledge.

That said, my contemporary, Yoga Teacher Richard Rosen, has also – like Yogani – written with clarity of many of the things that have come to me during my Pranayama practice, and Richard's books put many of these things into a helpful, unified, Yogic-overview context.

In <u>The Yoga of Breath</u>, (2002), and <u>Pranayama Beyond the Fundamentals</u>, (2006), Richard teaches the practice of Pranayama as taught by B.K.S. Iyengar, which differs from my approach. There are of course many schools of thought. What is important is that Richard knows what he is talking about.

"Skull-Shiner"

Kapalabhati is often translated as "skull shiner," but the term can be somewhat ambiguous, or can have multiple meanings.

The sinuses, your Third Eye Area, are cleared out, readied.

You may feel the skull tingle.

The entire crown of your head may feel luminescent, a "shining skull."

Beads of sweat may give you a shiny forehead. (With practice over time this sweating will become less or even non-existent in Kapalabhati and other Pranayama.)

On a higher level, your Sixth and Seventh Chakra areas, associated with the skull, may be opened up.

Or,

> Kapalabhati can open up/clear the <u>interior</u> of the skull wonderfully. You <u>feel</u> this. A luminescent interior skull. (I myself, perhaps just currently, vote for this as my preferred interpretation of the "skull shiner" effect.)

Post-Kapalabhati

Sit for a while after the practice…if only to recover.

After Kapalabhati notice where you are, right then, physically and emotionally. Notice how you feel. (It is helpful to do this after every Pranayama.) You might feel as though you are now up in your head, maybe in your Third Eye Area.

Ideally, when you come out of Kapalabhati you should feel more calm, quiet and even. The breath should have calmed down. You should feel more "grounded," in both senses of the word; that is, nicely, heavily down into the sitz-bones, and psychologically empowered/unfazed. Kapalabhati gives you confidence.

As mentioned above, you may well find that your Third Eye Area experiences some sort of activation. Regarding this, I believe I understand that Dr. Vasant Lad, one of the premier Ayurvedic practitioners in the United States, has indicated that the deeper meaning of Kapalabhati relates to an increase in cellular intelligence.

As you sit there you may experience Kevala Kumbhaka, the wonderful involuntary cessation for the breath. You just sit there, not breathing, and feeling great about it.

Take a Short Break Afterwards…

When you are done with your one minute's worth of Kapalabhati I suggest you <u>at the very least</u> take three full breaths before proceeding on to the next Pranayama. And I suggest that you consider taking a <u>one minute</u> break. Usually one minute means about ten breaths – each breath being one Inhale and one Exhale. Your system <u>needs</u> to recover.

SECRETS OF SUCCESSFUL PRANAYAMA

Notice if, after a few breaths, your shoulders naturally relax and drop down and/or your diaphragm relaxes. Both are pleasant feelings, and show you where you have been holding unconscious tension.

You may wish to repeat a simple Mantra like "Ahm-Sah" over and over as you sit there recovering. (See "Interim Mantras," below.)

You may also wish to keep the tips of your thumbs in the notch between the tips of your index and middle fingers. I feel that this particular Mudra will help you focus on your Third Eye Area.

Or transfer your thumb-tips to the tips of your middle fingers, to help focus on your Throat Chakra. Or to the tips of your ring fingers to focus on your Solar Plexus Chakra.

Any of these is a good thing for you to do as you sit there.

If you choose the Mudra that helps you to focus on the Third Eye Area, I suggest you might try with your thumb to gently, subtly, push the tip of your second finger more forward than your index finger. This helps brings attention forward in the skull.

Or… find a thumb tip to finger position that feels right to you.

…Or Take a Longer Break Afterwards

If it feels right just to sit there, don't go on until you get an inner cue to do so.

After Kapalabhati – or, in fact, after any of the Pranayama – feel free to just sit there and wait for something to kick in, and then, if something does, feel free to follow where it leads. You do not have to be in a hurry to go on to your next "scheduled" Pranayama. Really Good Things can happen to those who wait.

Interim Mantras

As you sit there after any Pranayama, sensing where you are Right Now and letting the breath recover somewhat, it is often quite beneficial to internally repeat a simple Mantra to yourself, so that your mind doesn't wander, and thus stealthily lead you away from the path you want to be on.

The Mantra is used to tamp down your brain's thinking.

Don't worry overly much about sticking to constant repetition of your Mantra, or even using one Mantra to the exclusion of all others at this point. The initial goal in Mantra use is not necessarily to stay in it. The goal is to follow the procedure of thinking it, inevitably losing it as the thinking mind tries to reassert itself, and then coming back to it when you realize that you've lost it. You are training yourself.

A "Curative Breath"

If you come out of Kapalabhati feeling, even very temporarily, a bit dizzy or light-headed, or nauseous or panicky, then you have gone too far. Scale back next time.

And, this time, to get rid of the feelings, do the curative mentioned previously:

> As you Inhale, press down strongly into your thighs with the back of your wrists. Then Exhale with a nose-mouth-nose sequence.
>
> That is: Exhale through your nose initially, then through the mouth for a bit in the middle of your Exhale, and then finish off the Exhale with your nose.

Doing this sequence <u>two times</u> should release any accumulated pressure. And should also make you feel nicely grounded and settled.

If your ears feel a little blocked up after Kapalabhati, (similar to what you might feel in an airplane), this nose-mouth-nose Exhale should help release the ears also.

Avoiding these types of discomfort is one of the reasons I advise you to count during Kapalabhati, (and during some of the other Pranayama). You want to establish, through trial and error, just how much you can do without going too far. You are then able to avoid such pitfalls.

Other Aspects of Kapalabhati

Phenomena

After Kapalabhati you may experience phenomena. You may in fact experience phenomena at any point during your Pranayama practice.

Nowadays I myself sometimes even go zooming off just after I sit down, before I even "do" anything except start to settle in. Apparently I have unconsciously pushed some sort of button, or my system has become so acclimated to the initial stimuli that it takes over on its own.

I would like to emphasize that, generally, you enjoy and go with a phenomenon, but <u>without trying to hold on to it</u>. If a phenomenon should happen, let it continue for as long as it wants, then let go and move on. <u>Do not</u> grab hold of it and try to cling to it. Because that blocks you:

> He who binds to himself a joy
> Doth the winged life destroy;
> But he who kisses the joy as it flies
> Lives in Eternity's sunrise.
>
> William Blake, "Eternity"
> (With thanks to D. Beale)

Students report all kinds of incredible phenomena. It seems to vary tremendously in each individual. Two quite common phenomena, however, are (1) a pleasant, "going-deeper" involuntary bobbing or swaying of the head and/or torso, and (2) "light shows" and/or colors.

Some students, sometimes quite unconsciously, bob or sway their heads and/or torsos forward and backward or from side to side. (I myself have spontaneously gone both directions). If something like that occurs, savor it – but if it feels like it will never end, then at some point you must consciously shut down the swaying or bobbing and move on.

This phenomenon of head bobbing seems to be a universal sign of a meditative state. You can <u>induce</u> it. Rolling the eyes back into the top of the head at any point during Pranayama or Meditation seems to be one thing that might help effectuate this.

If you get any sort of light show you won't want to end it, but it seems, in my experience at least, to end involuntarily, by itself. Colors vary with each student. And in each individual student, can vary in different sessions.

Phenomena Note: if you feel like you are floating away, losing yourself completely, and if you maybe even start to be afraid you might never come back, that you might inadvertently die – you might choose to rein yourself back in.

This however, for me, now, (because of my fear and my clinging), is not something for me to be teaching you about, but for me to be wondering about. A more experienced practitioner has assured me that I will indeed come back. (I asked him if I could tell them, on the other side, that he had given me his word about this.)

Keep well in mind: these phenomena are not goals. (In both senses of the word.)

Therapeutic Kapalabhati

If your nasal passages are blocked, (for example, as by a cold), you can use a gentle Kapalabhati to try to open them. But once they open, STOP. Don't go on to one minute or to 108 rounds. You can then try going on to Nadi Shodana, hopefully with some success.

Why not do "Bhastrika?"

Bhastrika, (the "Bellows Breath" or "Breath of Fire"), is closely related to Kapalabhati. It differs however in that it involves both a forceful Inhale and a forceful Exhale.

I choose to practice Kapalabhati instead for two main reasons. With Bhastrika, (sometimes "bastrika"), you are more likely to become hyperventilated than with Kapalabhati. And secondly, with Kapalabhati there is more benefit from alveolar ventilation than with Bhastrika. That is, in Kapalabhati more oxygen gets into the little sacs in the lungs where it is transferred into the blood stream.

That said, I do sometimes practice Bhastrika, in conjunction with Kapalabhati. When my Kapalabhati is going well, going quick and strong, I sometimes change it into Bhastrika and focus on how the air and energy flows wonderfully though my Throat Chakra Area and Third Eye Area.

And furthermore, I often experience, and you may find, that even without conscious effort you can be taken spontaneously by your body into an extremely quick Kapalabhati that then seems to change its character into a Bhastrika-like activity. This is especially true if you are going at a rate of well over 120 breaths per minute.

It's all good.

Finally, note that the phrase "Bellows Breath" is not only a description of the pumping-the-breath one does in Bhastrika, it is also a very good description what Kapalabhati may feel like when done well. I have in fact experienced two distinct, physical "bellows" feelings during Kapalabhati, which feelings are likely related.

The upper torso can feel like it's becoming a bellows – with the wider end at the mid-torso and the peak at the neck – squeezing air up into the head. You can sense this and run with the rhythm of it. It feels fabulous.

Or. It can feel like air, (or Energy), is being pumped into the Third Eye Area from right behind it, with a "bellows" type of pumping action.

Potent Effects

In sum. What do I mean by calling Kapalabhati a <u>potent</u> Pranayama? Two things.

In the short term – in the Pranayama session itself – Kapalabhati can get you "in" deep. That is, it can help get you <u>into</u>, or help get you <u>deeper</u> into, an altered state.

Secondly, in the bigger picture, quite simply, like most Pranayama, even if just practiced by itself, <u>Kapalabhati makes your life better</u>.

Preview

In Volume II, Intermediate Practices, I will discuss more of the nuances of Kapalabhati, as well as some more strenuous and potent variations that you can utilize as your practice advances.

Why all these Variations in the Pranayama?

Yes, you are being, and will be, introduced to number of options in almost every Pranayama.

Why didn't I just "Keep-It-Simple-Stupid?" After all, it's so much easier to say "Just do A, B and C and you're done."

Well, yes. Just so. A very good argument can be made for doing the same simple Pranayama over and over and over, all the time, and thus getting deeper and deeper and deeper into purification.

But then: what if you are missing out on something that might be even more potent for you? If you are not open to going to where you are led, or to exploring the possibilities that I or others bring to your attention, how do you know where your very best path lies?

And also… different people find that different things work for them.

So I am offering you a buffet.

Further, you yourself may well find that different options resonate with you at different stages of your progress in Pranayama. This is a reference book that can be consulted as you advance, in order to try out things that were perhaps hazy to you on your first read(s), but that might at a later point become more clear to you, have more real-life meaning for you.

If you do want simplicity, however, do find whatever works for you. (It is working if: <u>your life gets better.</u>) And concentrate on doing that, over and over.

Find your personal path. It's all good.

13

Nadi Shodana

The Basic Truth Behind It

Nadi Shodana, (Nah-dee Show-dah-nah), is a basic, major Pranayama practice.

Nadi means "Energy Channel." Shodana means "Cleanse." Nadi Shodana breathing is said to purify some major Energy channels in your body, and ready these channels for the flow of Energy in the deeper Pranayama that may follow in your practice session.

Two Types of Nadi Shodana

Nadi Shodana is often thought of as "Alternate-Nostril Breathing" and practiced in some "back-and-forth" manner. Some schools of thought, however, include "Single-Nostril Breathing," (breathing in and out through the same nostril), under its aegis. Some sources even describe Single-Nostril Breathing as Nadi Shodana, not as an alternative.

This chapter discusses the "Alternate-Nostril Breathing" mode. The "Single-Nostril Breathing" mode will be addressed in Volume II, Intermediate Practices.

Why Nadi Shodana is Important

Nadi Shodana helps you become, physically, "centered." It tends to "close down" the sides of your body and place you into the central line of your body. And you want this. It is empowering.

Along that central line, (roughly, up and down the spine), there is said to be a subtle "Central Energy Channel," which in Yogic terminology is called your "Sushumna." And indeed, once you have felt Energy going up and down the center of your body you will no longer question the existence of an "Energetic Body" on a different plane than your physical body.

Nadi Shodana prepares your Energy channels for you, before you try to bring Energy up, or up and down, them. It also prepares your body for Meditation by balancing Energies and quieting you down. It is therefore in one sense a preparatory step. (In another sense, all Pranayama, though of immense value in and of themselves, are "preparations" for Meditation.)

Nadi Shodana is very potent as a daily cleanser. With it – again, as with all Pranayama – you are removing psychic crud that can prevent you from linking up with (yoking to; "Yoga"), and flowing with, Universal Power.

If you have purified yourself regularly, you are then able to flow more in synch, more like clear water, not muddied or blocked. In this clear condition you don't lose/waste so much energy fighting the current. And it is so much better to flow downriver, with the Force, than to fight upstream. Your daily life can flow with fewer blockages, mirroring the increased flow of Energy in "you" and manifesting the body-mind-spirit connection.

Nadi Shodana's Importance is Recognized

Nadi Shodana and Kapalabhati (or Kapalabhati's brother, Bhastrika) are, to my knowledge, the "Big Two" – the two most widely-suggested Pranayama practices. Some sources and schools of Yoga just recommend

NADI SHODANA

one, or both, and nothing further. Every school I know of recommends Nadi Shodana in one form or another.

> "Variation is permissible … in the type of pranayama practised… Nadi Shodana Pranayama, however, should be practised daily."
>
> Yoga Teacher B.K.S Iyengar
> <u>Light on Yoga</u>, page 432

I personally have become more and more convinced that Iyengar is correct, that it is important to do some rounds of the "Alternate-Nostril Breathing" type of Nadi Shodana daily. The beneficial effects of Pranayama are much more likely to occur when this is done than when it is omitted.

One reason that Nadi Shodana is so often recommended may be that it can be considered, in its basic forms, a relatively easy Pranayama to do. There are other, more difficult Pranayama, which may perhaps get you "deeper" into things, but to which perhaps not as many people are willing, or able physically, to travel. And Nadi Shodana gives you a solid foundation for these.

But note that when you really get going into a long session of Nadi Shodana, it is of course <u>not</u> easy.

Because of its importance, this Guidebook will spend more time on Nadi Shodana and its variations than on any other Pranayama. This chapter will be divided into two sections:

1. Nadi Shodana – Basics
2. Nadi Shodana – Details

   Initial Positioning
   Your Inhale
   Your Retention
   Your Exhale
   Your Recovery

1. Nadi Shodana – Basics

The Breath

As a preliminary, Exhale (longishly) through both nostrils, then pinch (say) your right nostril shut with your right thumb. (Or your left nostril with your left thumb).

If you do shut your right nostril down, then:

1. Inhale through your open <u>left</u> nostril.
2. Pinch both nostrils closed. Hold your breath.
3. Open your <u>right</u> nostril, (letting go with your thumb), and Exhale through it.
4. Inhale through your now-open <u>right</u> nostril.
5. Pinch both nostrils closed. Hold your breath again.
6. Open your <u>left</u> nostril once again and Exhale through it.

This cycle of six "Stages" equals one "Round" of Alternate-Nostril Breathing.

Note that when you are just starting out in Pranayama you may need to omit, or may choose to omit, the "hold your breath" stage of the round and just do the Inhale and the Exhale, if that is your current capability. However:

Retention (holding your breath) is Important
Try to work up to it

Note that I am referring to a Retention after your Inhale. I do not advise beginners to hold their breath after the Exhale in Nadi Shodana. As I indicated previously, I consider this "Bahya Kumbhaka" a more advanced practice, and I think a lengthy Bahya Kumbhaka has some dangers.

NADI SHODANA

Important Note on Omitting the Retention

PREGNANT WOMEN can just Inhale and Exhale, without a Retention. My lay opinion is that you do not want to risk impeding the flow of oxygen to the fetus.

That said, one of my most headstrong, and physically strong, students did a full Pranayama practice up until the very week of her delivery, as well as a full Asana practice, which included, to my horror, right in front of my disapproving eyes, unsupported Scorpion Pose (an advanced forearm balance).

And then, snapping her fingers at me, she delivered a healthy and wonderful baby girl. ... I then Exhaled.

The point being: I have, obviously, little personal expertise in this particular area.

I have also read that menstruating practitioners should also just Inhale and Exhale without a Retention. I am somewhat skeptical of this because often these sources recommend little or no activity for menstruating women. (I have, obviously...)

Perhaps Related Note: Yoga, (and Pranayama), were for eons a male-only domain, (which is perhaps ironic nowadays).

Your Ratios

You need to decide what ratio of Inhale to Retention to Exhale you want to use. There are a myriad of possibilities. The easiest of all is a simple 1-1-2. That is, if you can count to, say, 10, as you Inhale, you would also Retain for 10, and then Exhale for 20.

Note that the longer Exhale makes the breath flow much more easily than does a simple 1-1-1- ratio. And that having your Exhale longer than your Inhale has calming qualities, which you are seeking.

You might like, for more benefit, to work up, <u>over time</u>, towards the much-lauded 1-4-2 ratio.

Symmetry

Strive towards complete symmetry between the activities of the two nostrils. Ideally your right nostril and left nostril Inhales, Retentions and Exhales should be exactly the same lengths of time in a round. That is, your right and left nostril Inhales are the same length as each other, your two Retentions are of equal length, and your right and left nostril Exhales are the same length.

Balance, Harmony and Flow are key words in both Pranayama and Yoga. And with symmetry in Nadi Shodana you achieve, at the least, Balance and Harmony.

"Continuous Rounds" versus "Rounds with Rests"

After the final Exhale of your initial round you may immediately begin another round with an Inhale through the same nostril out of which you have just Exhaled. And you may keep on going in that uninterrupted manner through more of these "Continuous Rounds."

Alternatively, you can do "Rounds with Rests." Here are two options you may choose:

<u>First Option</u>. After your first Exhalation, (Stage 3 above), you may just sit there for a while, breathing normally, hands in the lap, to recover somewhat. This is a Rest in the <u>middle </u>of a round. And then you may do another half-round, starting with an Inhale through your second nostril, (Stage 4 above). And then take another Rest break. And go on in that manner.

<u>Second Option</u>. Or you can perform a <u>full</u> Round, and then after your final Exhale, (Stage 6 above), sit and Rest, letting your breath recover. And then go on in <u>that</u> manner.

Both of these are easier than Continuous Rounds. And both are potent enough.

Many variations are of course available. You can do two or more Continuous Rounds, then have a Rest, and then do more Continuous Rounds. Or do a mixture of the First Option and Second Option Rounds with Rests. Or do a mix of Continuous Rounds and those Options.

The mind boggles... but, again, It's All Good.

How Many Rounds?

If over time you develop a strong Nadi Shodana practice, (i.e., your Inhale, Retention and Exhale are all very lengthy), my experience is that you can get good benefits from doing one round. However, other than in that circumstance, I suggest doing at least two or three Rounds. I personally consider two rounds an acceptable minimum. And I think four rounds is much better.

Why four rounds? First of all, and importantly, it keeps you going long enough to get better results from your Nadi Shodana. For one thing, the longer you practice Nadi Shodana in a session, the more your brain should quiet down. Which is a very good thing.

And there are two other, more minor considerations. As you become more advanced, four rounds enables you – if you switch hands after two rounds – to achieve symmetry. And even if you don't switch pinching hands, four rounds fits nicely with counting your rounds with your down hand: thumb-tip to first, second, third and fourth fingers equals four rounds.

Twelve Rounds. You can if you wish work up over time to a perhaps-maximum of twelve Continuous Rounds. Twelve Continuous Rounds is a Long Time! It is a long, slow, fascinating slog. It teaches patience and determination.

I myself have settled on twelve rounds for when I do a lengthy Nadi Shodana practice. Based on years of experimentation I feel it is quite potent in its "life-effects." And on the immediate level of the practice session itself, I find it is very likely to put me into a deep meditative state afterwards, and/or into breathing up and down my

Central Channel, which feels wonderful and is also, I firmly believe, desirable.

Note: if you are doing Nadi Shodana as part of a multi-Pranayama session, twelve rounds are doable only if your session is quite lengthy.

Why a <u>maximum</u> of twelve rounds? For one reason, because that number should allow you adequate time, in a session of some length, for the practice of other important Pranayama, while more than twelve might not.

And I note that the very experienced and deeply knowledgeable Yoga Teacher Baba Hari Dass similarly recommends starting with ten rounds, but also working up to a maximum of forty continuous rounds. However, his version of Nadi Shodana does not include Retentions. Therefore his 40 Inhales and 40 Exhales – of the same lengths – total out to what we might describe as a "work time" of 80. (80 times the length of your Inhale.) And if you instead use the "Twelve Rounds" technique suggested in this book with a 1-4-2 ratio, your "work time" will be a very similar 84. There thus appears, happily, to be some congruity.

2. Nadi Shodana: Details
Initial Positioning

Getting Ready to Inhale

Exhale calmly. Bring (say) your right hand up, palm towards your body, with your thumb poised for closing your right nostril down. I say "right hand" only because if you are right-handed it seems more natural to start that way. If you are left handed, or it seems more natural to use your left hand, use it.

You may want to use the same hand to start out with every time. It is one less thing to think about. And it is also then less likely that you will get lost, (yes, lost – the brain can get fuzzy), if you do go through several Nadi Shodana rounds.

An Inhaling Option: Begin with the Weaker Nostril

That said, in any given session you <u>may</u> want to start with your first Nadi Shodana Inhale coming up through that day's "weaker" nostril – (the one that is more "blocked," as determined by your previous "nostril testing") – and thus use your opposite hand as your Pinching Hand.

The reasoning behind this is this: if you start with the stronger nostril, the weaker nostril tends to get more quickly exhausted. This is because your breathing ability has been pre-depleted by the first-done stronger-nostril Inhale/Retention/Exhale work.

To say this again, but with different wording: if you start with the strong nostril, your respiratory system may be stressed/tired by the time you get to your weaker nostril, and thus your abilities with that second nostril may not be adequate for you to achieve the same numbers as you did with the first, stronger, nostril, and therefore will put you out of balance, out of harmony.

Keep in mind that a nostril can be also considered "weak" for your purposes if it is too <u>easy</u> to Inhale through it. If it is very easy to Inhale through it, it becomes – perhaps counter-intuitively – more difficult to Inhale through it for an extended period of time.

Starting with the weaker nostril may also be important because the weaker nostril is the one which tells you how deeply you can go in the breathing. So <u>its</u> limitations should limit you, in both your lengths and your ratios, as you go through your rounds.

For example, if you can only do, say, a 1-2-2 ratio with your weaker nostril, but you can do a 1-4-2 ratio using the stronger nostril, you should stick with a 1-2-2 because you want balance, harmony and symmetry.

In sum. As described previously, you may wish at the start of that day's session to test your nostrils to determine if one is weaker on the day. And if your testing does show you that one nostril is <u>dramatically</u> less open than the other, consider starting your Nadi Shodana with that less open nostril. Especially if you plan on doing many rounds.

If there is no great disparity, I'd say start with whichever side feels more natural.

Your Nose-Pinching Hand

Your <u>thumb</u> and your <u>ring finger</u> (or your <u>middle finger</u> if that feels better to you) are poised, like an open pliers, ready to pinch the nostrils shut.

Rest/push the tip of your thumb solidly into your cheekbone; this gives your arm a welcome steadiness. (With thanks to Martha Q. for this tip.)

Press the backs of the fingernails of your index and middle fingers, (if the ring finger is pinching), into the first knuckle-crease of your thumb. Press them, (and thus the thumb) towards your nose.

This helps to establish a tight lock. And, if these fingers stay in the air they tend to get in the way, or wander, or even want to scratch the nose.

Your Lap Hand

Likewise, with the very same pressure, press the fingernails of your lap-hand index and middle fingers into that hand's thumb knuckle-crease. (With thanks to Chris P. for this tip.)

These equal pressures, (nostril pinching hand fingernail pressure and lap hand fingernail pressure), are very helpful - they bring you into a nice balance that greatly enhances your abilities in Nadi Shodana, including your ability to stay in an extended Retention.

Pinching-Hand Arm Position 1: For Many Rounds

When you start your breathing I suggest you let your upper arm fall just slightly out to the side away from your body. If it is clamped in tight to the chest it can impede a full inhale.

However, I do not advise taking it too far away, nor holding it out parallel to the floor – it takes too much energy to hold it out there for an extended period of Nadi Shodana. Further, holding the arm parallel to the floor can put more force into your "thumb clamp" and less into your "finger clamp," which may upset balance, (but see below).

An Alternative Pinching-Hand Arm Position: For a Low Number of Rounds

If you are doing, say, four rounds or less then you can try lifting your pinching arm elbow up into the air to approximately parallel to the floor, and with your elbow forward rather than directly out to the side from your shoulder.

Because you are doing a relatively small number of rounds the arm should not get excessively tired; and there are two advantages to this position.

1. The thumb can be pressed much more firmly into the nostril, thus establishing a (desirable) tighter lock; and, to help maintain that:
2. Instead of using just your ring or middle finger to pinch your other nostril closed you can use your first two fingers, or your middle and ring fingers, one higher up the nostril than the other or else piggy-backing. This allows a more complete closure; and, with the arm raised, more pressure can be applied on this nostril also, resulting in a firm lock on both sides.

That said, I do not do this. I am accustomed to Pinching Position 1.

Face Position

Your chin is slightly tucked down. I strongly advise this. For one thing, this chin position enhances/induces the relaxation responses you seek. For another it relieves physical tension in the neck/throat area caused by the practice.

But do not go further down and establish a Chin Lock.

Your head may tend to turn slightly in the direction of the pinching hand. Be aware of this tendency and correct yourself if necessary. You want symmetry. Thus you want your nose to feel like it is pointing straight ahead.

The Body

Keep the whole body alive, especially the pinching arm, which often tends towards lassitude or deadness.

Your Inhale

Even before you do your first Nadi Shodana Inhale, you can enhance the practice more by making sure you take a deep preliminary Inhale, and then a long preliminary Exhale.

Then pinch your thumb-side nostril shut with your thumb and take your first long Inhale.

It is <u>key</u> to keep your Inhale <u>slow</u> and <u>controlled</u> at the <u>start</u> of it. Concentrate on this.

Start the Inhale in your lower body and bring it up, diagonally, into your upper back, behind the heart. <u>Not higher</u>. (See below.)

As you slowly and gradually Inhale, expand your rib cage to create more space in order to allow more air in. Fill your rib cage with air. Expand. Try to fill your upper back ribs.

Later on in your round you will Inhale into your second nostril with the same length and intensity as you just did with your first nostril. Resist any temptation to Inhale more deeply into your second nostril. Aiming as always for symmetry and balance, you Inhale equally into both nostrils.

Using a Portion of the Nostril

You should try to make your Inhale as <u>thin</u> and <u>narrow</u> and <u>reedy</u> as possible, in order to make it last as long as possible. To make it long and thin and narrow, experiment with Inhaling either through the upper portion, (the roof), of your nostril, or the lower portion, (the floor), or at the inside or outside wall of the nostril.

Or try to get even more specific than that. For my left nostril I often use the "outside corner of the nostril floor" and for my right nostril I usually use the "inside wall" or the "outside floor."

Your optimum location may depend on the condition of the nostril at the time of your specific practice, and can vary a great deal. See what works for you.

These are of course more advanced considerations, to be tried out after you have the basics down pat.

Don't "Fill to the Brim" or "Round Off" the Inhale

Do not Inhale to the absolute maximum you are able to do. This creates too much pressure on the system. You want to fill to, as it were, just below your brim.

So. Don't bring the Inhale up your back and up over your shoulders to your front, trying to ultra-fill yourself. Again: Inhale up to the level of the heart. Not into the throat or nose; that creates too much pressure/stress. Your shoulders shouldn't hunch during the Inhale. You might even want to consciously drop your shoulders to avoid rounding off your Inhale.

Rounding off often occurs if you have to rush your Inhale.

If it feels like you are "sprinting" in order to get enough air in, it means your prior Exhale was too long.

Push the Inhale into the Back into the Spine

Once you have Inhaled continue to push the air back into your spine. This is important. It helps solidify everything.

Try Not to "Surge"

In your later rounds especially – when your Inhale is more difficult because you have been, effectively, starving your system of the oxygen it thinks it needs – the Inhale tends to "surge" towards the end of the Inhale.

One quite effective way to counter this: as you get towards the tail end of your Inhale, apply more pressure with the thumb or finger that is pressing the opposite nostril shut.

If, in any event, you feel you must surge, just surge the breath up into the chest, but not to the throat, to avoid untoward pressure and stress.

Wing Your Arms

If you are having trouble Inhaling for as long a count as you would like, as you reach the middle of your Inhale start slowly raising both your elbows up into the air out to the sides, like a bird expanding its wings. Continue to slowly do this until you reach your full Inhale. I believe it helps expand your lung capacity.

Count

Count as you Inhale. You will note that silent counting is an integral part of many of the Pranayama in this Guidebook. I don't believe this is merely a misplaced emphasis on exactitude. It serves to tell you exactly where you are in a Pranayama. And I feel it also furthers your progress towards two worthy goals:

1. It helps you to establish your "Edge," that is, how deeply (and thus potently) you can do the Pranayama to extract the maximum possible benefit without any deleterious, stressful side effects. Or at the least it can help you to establish where your "comfort zone" is.
2. It occupies the mind, thus helping keep it calm and relatively unthinking, a desirable condition during the Pranayama. Thinking destroys Pranayama.

Your Retention

Chin Lock

You may wish to experiment doing Nadi Shodana with or without a Chin Lock. There is no need for a Chin Lock if you are not doing a Retention.

Establishing a Chin Lock (Jalandhara Bandha) immediately after you hit the top of your Inhale will help you stay in your Retention longer. It is very helpful to swallow after reaching the top of your Inhale, just before you apply your Chin Lock.

You may, after your reach the apex of your Inhalation elongate your neck, then take your chin out and then down into the notch of your throat, and, as you do so, lift your chest up into the chin. Get tight.

Hold yourself in that position, keeping things locked up, during your entire Retention.

It is important to bring the chest <u>up</u> into the Chin Lock so that Energy can rise up the system to the appropriate degree. This is perhaps not as important now, in Nadi Shodana, as it is later, when you want to consciously bring Energy up the body, but I advise that you get in the habit of lifting up the chest at this point.

To establish a really deep Chin Lock, shrug both your shoulders up as high as you can, then take your chin down into your neck notch. Then release your shoulders back down again. Your chin will be tighter into your chest.

Another helpful hint is to push your chin <u>way out</u> and then bring it back down and into your throat.

Your Chin Lock may lead you quite nicely into also establishing a Mini Belly Lock, (a soft "Uddiyana Bandha").

The Nose-Pinch

Using my ring finger along with my thumb is, to me, just right. Using my thumb and my little finger tends to close my arm down. Using my thumb and first finger puts my hand at an awkward angle.

And, for me, using the middle finger to pinch does not close my nose at a good angle. However, many of my students seem to prefer it to the ring finger. So maybe it's just me. On the other hand, using the ring finger is what many schools advise.

An Alternative Pinching-Hand Position

Some people have been trained to put their first two fingers onto the Third Eye Area of the forehead, usually somewhere between and above the eyebrows. This doesn't work for me. Experiment and find your own comfort zone.

The Pinch Itself

There are three separate, subtle, force-lines for your pinching.

First of all, of course, you pinch your nostrils IN towards the center line of your nose. You should do this at a position that is relatively high up – near the cartilage, even nudging into it, rather than lower down on the lobe. Because this creates a more solid, useful, pinch.

Second, your pinching fingers also pull, slightly and subtly DOWN on your nostrils, or else your nose can feel uncomfortably full of air during your Retention.

Third, your pinching fingers should also push, slightly and subtly INTO your skull. For one thing, this helps keep the body erect.

These three forces (pinch in, pull down, and push into) work best for me. The down-pull and push-into combine to create a diagonally directed force both down and into the skull, and I find this somehow helpful.

Retain up to Four Times as Long as Your Inhale

Try to hold your breath for at least as long as your Inhale. If you can hold for longer – up to <u>four</u> times as long – that's much better. Retain long, but to your own capability, and not, I suggest, more than four times as long as your Inhale. I think longer than that is inappropriate for beginners.

If your Retention does in fact approach or achieve four times the length of your Inhale, realize that the last bit of your Retention (say the last quarter of it) may be difficult to master. It becomes more about inner calm and willpower.

Counting During Retention

Try to count during your Retention at the same speed with which you counted during your Inhale. You want this in order to establish the ratios you desire between the lengths of your Inhale, Retention and Exhale.

That said, it is tricky to do this same-speed counting. For some reason the speed of your counting during your Inhale usually differs from your speed in counting during your Retention. It may be much faster during the Inhale, or slower.

For example, for years I did a 1-4-2 <u>count</u> – thus trying to achieve a 1-4-2 <u>ratio</u> in real time. But then my students actually timed my counts a few times. My Retention – with this <u>four</u> count – was in reality <u>seven</u> times as long as my Inhale, not four times as long.

I experimented more at home. They were right.

What to do? I rather liked the feel of my bogus "four times as long." I played with cutting it back. And this certainly made extended rounds of Nadi Shodana easier.

So. What do I advise you to do? I think the ancients probably didn't have stopwatches. Did they rely on their internal and perhaps "bogus" count to arrive at a 1-4-2 ideal? Or did their guru time them externally.

Am I to advise you to do a "four times as long count," or work for real-time "four times as long?"

Damn my students. I hate it when they do that. I was so comfortable.

Okay. I'll straddle the fence. I don't see any harm in either method. If you can time yourself now and then and establish what your "count" should be in order to get to a "real-time" four-times-as-long Retention, feel free to use that count. Or continue to use your "bogus' count, but now not feeling quite as bad about the difficulty of it.

(The best of both worlds.)

I personally have decided to stay with my extra-long count, probably because I'm so habituated to it. And then, also, when I am doing a long number of rounds and things are getting tough, I can scale back my count, without excessive guilt.

Voluntary Head Bobbing

One effortless way to make your Retention longer, and thus more potent, is by voluntarily taking your head, or your head and your torso, into a slight forward-and-backward bobbing. I myself bob my head, often in time with the rhythm of my count, and I heartily recommend it. Try a Retention without the bobbing and then try one with bobbing. The difference may be considerable. Again, I myself do this bobbing every single Retention, as do many of my more advanced students.

Pressure in Retention

If pressure or tension builds up too much during Retention, open your finger (but keep your <u>thumb</u> tight against your nostril) and let a little puff or blurp of air out through the nose. Or perhaps a little involuntary swallow will occur. Or both the <u>puff</u> and the <u>swallow</u>. Then continue. You may do this as many times as necessary in Nadi Shodana; but it may be an indication that you have Inhaled too much or are trying to Retain past your current capacity.

If things get too stressful in general in Nadi Shodana: <u>Stop</u>. Breathe normally a few times to let the stress dissipate. Then try again if you wish.

Your Mind

It is important to be mentally "soft" and unthinking during your Retention.

You can if you wish pick a point in the body or outside it to focus your mind on.

<u>Shoulder Focus</u>. I suggest you might want to use the area between your shoulder blades, as I have found it to be best for me.

<u>Focus Out in Front of the Chest</u>. Or it may be better for you to put your closed eyes (and perhaps your mind) just softly, lightly down into the <u>air</u> in front of your chest.

Looking slightly down with your closed eyes, and with your chin tilted down, into the space in front of your torso helps establish a longer, calmer Retention. But looking further down, into the chest itself, seems to me to create too much tension.

The flow of the eyes looking down in front of the body also serves to balance the flow of the Inhale up to a Retention in the upper back.

<u>Scanning</u>. Or, if you wish to, you can multi-task your mind, occupying it so it doesn't go into stray thinking:

  (1) Focus on your count – and then:
  (2) Focus on keeping your chest big – and then:
  (3) Focus on keeping your eyes and mind down in front of you.
  (4) Focus on keeping all the pressing of the fingers in your two hands equal.
  (5) Focus on belly subtly in and up, heart and throat subtly down.

You can continue to constantly scan between these foci, (or some of them) (and in any order) (or whatever works for you), both to remind yourself what to do and to avoid other thoughts. The scanning acts as kind of a pseudo-Mantra.

If the mind does wander during Retention? Remember: this can degrade or even destroy the practice. Repeat <u>something</u> over and over. Try to squelch the wandering.

> Note Well: despite all the focus in this chapter on physical technique, the most important thing in Alternate Nostril Breathing is your <u>Intent</u>.

Finish in Control

At the end of your Retention clench your diaphragm slightly, if necessary, so that you are not forced to start your Exhale with an uncontrolled explosion, or with a quick, panicky start, but are instead in control.

Your Exhale

After your Retention open up the nostril you had originally clamped shut with your <u>thumb</u> during your Inhale. Keeping your other nostril clamped shut with your clamping finger, Exhale out through the now-opened nostril for <u>twice as long</u> as your Inhale.

These instructions are of course reversed for the second Exhale of a round. Your thumb stays clamped and your finger releases its nostril.

Note that your Exhale is your "canary in the mine." Failure to achieve a twice-as-long Exhale tells you that your Inhales and/or Retentions are too long. If this twice-as-long Exhale proves difficult, reduce the length of your Retention. If it is still difficult after that, reduce the length of your Inhale.

One way to make your Exhale last twice as long – if your Inhale has been very long – is to try at the start of your Exhale to let the air seep slowly, even almost imperceptibly, out of your nostril. Then continue to Exhale, so slowly that there is hardly any air at all coming out of your nostril. And at the end of the Exhale you may use a tiny bit of sustained pushing force, if necessary clenching your torso, to keep the outflow going.

If you start to feel <u>panicky</u> towards the end of your Exhale, try loosening your throat and see if that helps you make it to twice-as-long. And then make sure you lessen your Retention a bit next time.

If you are hunching over at the end of your Exhale, in order to try to force that last bit of air out, you are trying too hard.

Don't Burst Out of the Gate

Again, keep control of your Exhale from the very start. Use your muscular strength in the area of your diaphragm to make sure you begin the process slowly.

Counting

Count as you Exhale. Use the same counting speed as your Inhale and Retention counting.

Even Out the Flow

Just as you tried to make your <u>Inhale</u> thin and long and narrow, you want to do the same thing on your <u>Exhale</u>. It may help, as mentioned above, to be a little bit forceful with your Exhale – especially towards the end of it – if this helps you to maintain a long, long, even flow.

Staying High & Dropping Down

It can be helpful if you do not let your <u>eyes, cheekbones, chest</u> or <u>brain</u> sag down as you Exhale, especially towards the end of the Exhale when things may be becoming a bit forced and panicky. Instead, it may be helpful to consciously lift these, very subtly, <u>up</u>.

Do however drop your shoulders down in order to make things go more smoothly. The shoulders tend to clench and rise up as things get difficult.

You might note that these activities, when combined, can contribute to an arching of the back. And indeed, consciously arching during every Exhale, (the opposite of hunching over), is both a good way to elongate your Exhale and to not get all slumpy.

Another good way to elongate your Exhale is raise your elbows slowly upwards as you Exhale.

Once again, in all this, you are balancing up and down forces.

And again, keep in mind that these are all very subtle actions.

Exhale to Rock Bottom, Then Swallow

It is important to determine your Edge, that is, how long an Exhale you can achieve without distress. You want to identify, over time, the maximum number to which you can ordinarily count during your Exhale. You may then aim to Exhale to that number, or near it, each time – to what you have determined is your Rock Bottom Exhale. Thus you stay in your established Comfort Zone.

Once you have reached your Rock Bottom Exhale number, (or a lesser number if you can't reach it), you swallow.

You swallow because when you do so it brings about a small, involuntary, further Exhalation. And more so because this further Exhale sets up your Inhale more perfectly, making the transition into it easier. It feels like a graceful swooping action, down at the end of the Exhale and then up into your Inhale. It also helps relieve any tension that builds up during the practice.

Regarding swallowing: if your throat is catching excessively and /or you are swallowing a lot during Nadi Shodana, try lower numbers, (i.e., don't go as long on your Inhales, Retentions and Exhales.) And try to quiet your mind more. Or swallow twice in a row at the end of your Exhale rather than just once. Swallowing twice in a row might be especially helpful during the earlier rounds of Nadi Shodana.

Note that this swallow at the end of your Exhale can also act as another "canary in the mine." If your swallow is decreased or almost non-existent, then you need to dial things back, trying lower numbers for your Inhales and Retentions. You are trying too hard.

Start Back Calmly

See if you achieve a brief sense of complete calm at the end of your Exhale, so that you can begin Inhaling again without any sense of panic, with no need to gasp.

Your Recovery

After Nadi Shodana, sit there with your eyes closed and just breathe for a while. Take at least three or four breaths before proceeding. Taking ten breaths should give you about a one minute recovery, which you might find to be, normally, adequate.

It might prove helpful to make your first Inhale and Exhale of the ten deep and full, to help you back to tranquility. And you might want to let this Exhale be out through your mouth. Especially if you need to relax tension: take an Exhale or two out through your mouth.

Observe

See what, if anything, is going on during your recovery.

Your back may arch and your chest open, creating a wonderful opening/ blossoming in the heart area.

You may notice how wonderfully quiet and long the spaces after your Exhales are now. Let these spaces grow if you wish.

Phenomena may kick in.

You might feel a centralization of the Energy of the body. Nadi Shodana should have to some extent balanced out the Energies on (simplistically) the right and left Energy channels of the body, and thus made you more aware of/put you more into your central line. The sides of the body may feel like they have closed down. This is not insignificant.

Whether or not anything occurs, do notice the length of your Exhales, and also the length of the space after your Exhale and before your next Inhale. A lengthening of either of these two things is an indicator of the quieting and calming that Pranayama should induce.

Mudra in Recovery

Immediately after you have completed the Pranayama, you may wish to find and take a Mudra which is associated with your upper-body Chakras. You can put your thumb-tips onto the tips of your first fingers; first and second fingers; second fingers; or two middle fingers. Find what feels right to you, at that particular moment in time, and stay seated with your hands in that Mudra.

I suggest that you may well find the Heart Chakra Mudra – thumb tips to the notch between the tips of the middle and ring fingers – to be most satisfying.

Mantra in Recovery

You may wish to repeat, silently to yourself, "Ahm" on your Inhale and "Sah" on your Exhale, or some other simple Mantra during this quiet-time recovery period. I advise against a more complex Mantra here. I don't think the mind can wrap itself around it at this point.

Ujjayi in Recovery

You may be taken involuntarily in to Ujjayi Breathing, (discussed in Chapter 16). Or you may if you wish begin to do it voluntarily. If so, it should be feel natural, and good.

Discovering Your Central Line

Again, Nadi Shodana is designed in part to close down the sides of your body and put you into the center line of your body. You feel "centered."

If you wish to induce an appreciation of an approximation of your "central channel," as you sit there after Nadi Shodana lightly and quickly tap your Third Eye Area with a fingernail 10-15 times. Then lightly and quickly draw a line with that fingernail from your hairline, in the middle of your forehead, down the center of your body to just above the genitals.

Then tap again with a fingernail from your other hand, and draw another line.

See what happens.

When you do this tapping and drawing you may feel some sort of central line in your body. (You may feel it as a cold line).

Discovering Your Third Eye Area

Your Third Eye Area is located between the eyebrows (or slightly above them) and back into the head. To try to find it with closed eyes: hover a pointed finger over that general area, then go up and down with the finger in the air just in front of your forehead, searching. See if your body talks to you.

See if you can physically experience an area, perhaps about the size of an egg.

Feel, perhaps, power... or intensity.

You may also try to discover other Chakras by tapping. Tap your Third Eye. Then tap your other Chakras. See if you become more aware of them.

A Relevant Side Trip into Meaning: Sixth Chakra

> The "Sixth Chakra" is often called the Third Eye Chakra. And, in my experience, and in the experience of some of my students, the "Third Eye" is not a metaphor. When "deep" you may see a human eye looking back at you. In my experience thus far this appears in conjunction with peak spiritual occurrences. Note well: this is not a construct, nor an hallucination. It is an eye. Period.

"Tunnel" Vision

As you sit there, you may experience, as another "peak" type of experience: a sort of tunnel-like vision may develop or coalesce, perhaps with some sort of vision at the end of the tunnel. This tunnel has been said to be a Gateway.

Another Relevant Side Trip: Meaning of the Sixth Chakra

The Sanskrit name for what is most often called the "Third Eye Chakra" is "Ajna." It is pronounced "ugh-neeyah" and can be translated as "Command" or "Command and Control." Not because it commands or controls the other chakras. But because it is the portal or gateway through which we can receive directions, "commands" or insights from Universal Power. It is thus well worth cultivating, and perhaps why so much attention is directing at bringing Energy up, specifically, to it.

The "Sri Yantra," (a geometric design, which has many variations), can be said to be a symbolic representation your Central Channel ("Sushumna"). But likewise the Sri Yantra symbolically portrays – almost perfectly in my experience – this tunnel, which may be thought of as a continuation, out into space in front of your eyes, of the Sushumna.

Regarding the perfection of this portrayal: when I first saw a Sri Yantra design I exclaimed to myself "My God!" (Actually it was something way more earthy than that.)

A sample Sri Yantra is on the front cover of this Guidebook.

Misc.

As in Kapalabhati, do not distress the nostrils.

As in Kapalabhati, pushing the balls of the feet into the floor straightens the body, (and helps Energy to rise). For a very helpful balancing effect learn to push your feet into the floor with the exact same pressure as you are pressing your fingernails into your thumb knuckle-creases.

If you are very pinched for time, or just want a quick calming or quieting down, just do some Nadi Shodana by itself.

If pressure builds up, or you accumulate excess saliva in your mouth, stop momentarily, swallow, do a deep breath in and out, and then go back into your sequence.

Nadi Shodana is marvelous for alleviating headaches. Including migraines. Do it when you feel one coming on. Or when you are in the throes.

Summary:
Kapalabhati & Nadi Shodana

Again, these two practices might be considered to some extent to be preliminaries, readying your system – both during each individual practice and over time – for the other more rigorous active Pranayama and Energy Work that is necessary to practice in order to experience the full effect of what Yoga has to offer.

The flip side of this, however, is that both Kapalabhati and Nadi Shodana are potent enough, in and of themselves, to remain a part of your daily practice <u>forever</u>.

So. I think that if you are a complete beginner you would be well advised to concentrate on getting solid in <u>them</u> first. You might even be well advised to spend weeks or even months getting comfortable with the basics of these two Pranayama, (and Ujjayi breathing), before moving on into different variations of them, and then on to other Pranayama. That, however, takes some restraint.

Why all this Stressful Breathing & Non-Breathing?

You will have noticed that in many of the Pranayama I encourage you to extend the limits of your Inhales, Exhales, Retentions and Suspensions, utilizing techniques that are stress-producing.

Briefly, one theory behind this is that all this stressing of your body by depriving it of oxygen forces your individual cells to learn to adapt to the stress. They learn how to function better in these abnormal situations; they modify their structure, enabling them to hold more Energy within themselves. They become better, stronger, <u>to your benefit</u>.

And, to restate this in more detail, the stressing is aimed at:

Cellular Bliss for Life Extension and Anti-Aging

The physical aspects of Yoga were perhaps in part designed to give the ancient Yogis a healthy body so they could live long enough to advance spiritually as far as they possibly could.

How can Yoga increase life-span and keep the body young?

One "Yogic-scientific" explanation offered pertains to the effect of Yoga on the individual cells of our bodies. When our <u>muscles, glands</u> and <u>organs</u> are stressed during an Asana and/or Pranayama practice that is sustained over an extended period of time, our cells react to the stress. They learn how to function better in these abnormal situations; they modify their structure by absorbing new nutrients not ordinarily required and by modifying their excretory system.

These two modifications (improving the supply of nutrients and helping remove toxic cellular waste) enable the cell to hold more energy within it. The cell is now a better cell, ("blissful," if you will), and can devote more energy to the constructive "anabolic" process rather than the destructive, aging "catabolic" process.

14

Agni Sara

The Basic Truth Behind It

Kapalabhati and Nadi Shodana have begun the opening and cleansing of your Energy Channels and helped to center you. And have, in my opinion, worked the upper body. Now, with two further "Energy-Awakening" Pranayama you may attempt to purify the lower torso. And also, perhaps, to help further awaken Energy there that you wish to flow through your channels.

I myself think of these two activities – Agni Sara and Asvini Mudra – as "Pranayama-Kriyas" because they involve non-breath physical movement.

Agni Sara is, basically, belly-pumping after an Exhale. It is an introductory form of a Pranayama-Kriya called Nauli, (belly-churning), which is discussed in Volume II. The two are very closely related techniques, but they may have different after-effects for you.

The Set-Up

Because you are working in the area of the Second Chakra, in the lower abdomen, you may find it helpful to put your hands into the Second Chakra Mudra, that is, with your thumbs-tips in the notches between the tips of your ring and little fingers.

This may help make your pumping easier and last longer. As might rotating your palms diagonally inward as they rest on your thighs, so that they are more facing towards the lower abdomen.

Having done that, you preliminarily:

1. Exhale normally and then Inhale <u>big</u>.
2. Swallow and then Establish your Chin Lock.
3. Exhale out, <u>long and slow</u>, through your nose.

Do Not Do a Full Exhale

You want to Exhale long, but not too long. So, before practicing Agni Sara, you should try to get a feel for your normal maximum Exhale count. Do so by practicing Dirga Rechaka, that is, slowly Exhaling for as long as you can after a big Inhale.

Then, having established what your maximum number is, when you practice Agni Sara don't Exhale ultra-completely to that number. That would hamper the Pranayama. Instead just go to perhaps about two-thirds of the way there.

For example: if you can Exhale to a 60-count, just go to around 40 instead. If you do your full 60 you will be too depleted to get good results. My trials and, mostly, my errors, have led me to recommend this "about two-thirds" figure.

Or you may test various Exhale numbers over time in order to find the one which seems allow you to achieve the maximum number of quality belly pumps, and utilize it. For example, I myself have found that a 40-count Exhale enables me to perform a <u>significantly</u> higher number of quality pumps than does, say, a 50-count Exhale.

Notice that I say "quality" pumps. The goal is not to do as many pumps as possible. It is to awaken and send Energy.

And now:

> 4. When you have completed your Exhale, <u>swallow</u> – in order to get that little involuntary Exhalation that follows – and then, immediately...

The Pumping

> 5. Pump your <u>lower abdomen</u> in and out for as long as you can, without Inhaling.

Whereas in Kapalabhati you focus on jerking the <u>solar plexus</u> in, here you focus on pumping your <u>belly</u>, lower down than that. Think of it as the belly-button area if you wish, but I believe the area being worked is below the level of the belly-button, in the area of the Second Chakra, at the level, for women, of the ovaries.

Try to have your belly do the work. Try to not to let your shoulders move forward and back as you pump. In this regard it may be initially useful to sit in a chair that has a back, and to sit so that the back of the chair is pressing into your back. This helps stabilize your upper body and keeps the Pumping contained as much as possible in your belly.

If your throat starts to click that means that air is coming in. Make your Chin Lock tighter. If your throat continues to click, Stop. It is difficult to maintain a tight Chin Lock as you pump. Don't worry about it. But it is very helpful to keep your chin down.

Pump slowly or pump quickly, but always with a <u>fluid belly</u>. Get into Rhythm. Keep your diaphragm and belly and soft.

Keep your mind soft also, with the mind casually observing the fluidity of the belly. Put your mind into your belly. Try for a belly as fluid as a belly dancer.

Soft mind, soft belly. Calm mind, calm belly.

As the belly works, try to keep the rest of your body as calm as a statue, and to keep your mind as calm and blank as the mind of a statue.

Other keys to Pumping for a long time, (which is what you want), are to perhaps be in the whole body rather than a specific point, and to be balanced.

As you pump, you may want to push your feet gently into the floor. Don't curl your toes.

Other Versions

Note that this slow or quick pumping of the belly is different than the very slow "Agni Sara" Pranayama often taught. And note also that the same "Agni Sara" name is used, depending on the Yogic school doing the teaching, for other breathing/movement variations related to the tummy area.

The many variations of Agni Sara are also often taught standing up with the knees bent and the torso hunched over with the hands resting on the thighs or knees. This is a good way to do it, but I do not utilize it here because I do not wish you to relinquish your upright spine and lean that far forward as you sit in your chair, nor to stand up, coming in and out of your sitting pose. I think it is distracting.

You can however, if you wish, mimic this standing version by leaning your torso forward as you sit there, and placing your hands on your knees. Again, I don't necessarily advise this, nor do it, because I think that here, sitting in your chair, it is an unnecessary postural complication, despite the fact that you may be able to get deeper into an Uddiyana Bandha, (Belly Lock), in this leaning-forward position. I personally am more enamored, here, with vigorous Pumping.

Count Your Pumps

Count as you go. Do so in order to establish over time how many pumps you can do without stress, and without gasping when you come out. This way you will know when to stop. Your maximum will improve with time. Over the months and years your respiratory system and abdominal muscles will strengthen, and your abilities will increase, perhaps dramatically.

But do not focus your mind on trying to reach a predetermined number of pumps. As soon as you focus on a goal you seem to lose the ability to reach it. I think this may possibly be a result of the energy expended because of the mental tension involved in a perceived "must do" situation.

If you do count, instead of making the mind calm and blank, it is important to make it calm by focusing with purity on your count. Not on the total number you may wish to reach, which is a mental stressor, but the number(s) you are actually counting. Be solely in the Ones, Twos, Threes, Etc. This yields dividends.

How Many Rounds?

My personal opinion is that there are diminishing returns after doing two rounds of Agni Sara. Most often my practice includes just one, as it takes me into a nice calm where I want to reside for a while.

Recover

When it is right for you to do so – before things get overly stressful – Inhale, and go to normal breathing and Just Sit.

You may want to do "Your Curative," mentioned earlier, if needed after you have finished. It can be especially helpful after Belly Pumping.

Holding the Breath

The breath often seems to want to stop after Agni Sara. It can thus go by itself into involuntary "Kevala Kumbhaka" non-breathing. Or you yourself can just hold it voluntarily. Or you can hold it and while doing do so practice Asvini Mudra, (discussed in the next chapter).

Being in Your Third Eye Area

After you finish Agni Sara, you may wish to put yourself up into your Third Eye Area. And Be There.

Focusing yourself in your Third Eye Area after Agni Sara is a good thing to do. It is a good place to be. Many Pranayama practices are designed to take you up and locate you there.

Why is being in the Third Eye Area such a good thing? Because it takes you deep and keeps you there. Because it allows things to happen. Because you want your Energy to come UP, and being in the Third Eye Area helps draw it up.

And more.

<u>Involuntarily</u>. You may not have to <u>try</u> to put yourself up in the Third Eye Area, but just let yourself be taken there.

I believe that Agni Sara is very good for putting you involuntarily into your Third Eye Area; it may make it relatively easy for you to access the Area and stay there.

So wait and see if, at some point after you finish – even if you have not taken yourself "up" – you do go "up" involuntarily.

You may find that placing your thumb-tips on the notches between the tips of your index and middle fingers will assist you in this.

<u>Voluntarily</u>. You may try to actively take yourself up into your Third Eye by going almost immediately into Ujjayi Breathing. (Ujjayi Breathing is discussed later, in Chapter 16.)

By itself Ujjayi can both help take you up into the Third Eye Area or help keep you there. You may make your first Inhale as you complete your Agni Sara an Ujjayi Inhale up the central line of your body to your Third Eye Area. And then you may continue with Ujjayi, with your focus on your Third Eye Area.

Being in Your Throat Area, or…

Alternatively, you might wish to push your thumb-tips strongly against your middle fingertips and be in your Throat Chakra area (which I personally identify as not being in the upper throat but more or less at the notch between the collar-bones). This seems to bring calm and power, post-Agni Sara.

Or… find a thumb to finger position that seems right to you and see where your consciousness wants to settle in your body.

Constricted Breathing

Notice the degree of calm you may be feeling after Agni Sara.

If you have been at this type of practice for a while, Agni Sara might put you a bit closer to Sushumna Breathing – a subtle, deep-core type of breathing, a breathing-without-breathing kind of thing.

> [The yoga pose Mahamudra] freezes all the normal respiratory movements out of the body cavity….All in all the body is forced to find another, unusual way to breathe…something deep in the core must mobilize via new pathway. That pathway is commonly referred to in yogic literature as susumna – the central channel."
>
> Yoga Teacher L. Kaminoff
> Yoga Anatomy, p 115

The pumping of the lower abdomen in Agni Sara stirs up, stimulates and awakens the Energy that resides at the base of the spine. The work is thus helpful in enabling that Energy to rise upward, as you want it to.

A Relevant Side Trip:

Meaning of the Second Chakra

> The Sanskrit name of the second-lowest Chakra in the body – located in the lower abdomen – is "Swadisthana." This is often translated as "One's Own Abode."

The meaning of this was a mystery to me for quite a while. Many translators utilize a sexual/womb/ creativity angle, (according to their own bent), in describing the Chakra. However, as I now have come to understand it, the name is better translated as "The Abode of the One."

To my mind this is a reference to Kundalini, the name for a portion of the indivisible, basic (i.e., "One") Energy. This Kundalini reserve of Energy is said to reside at the base of the spine, in front of the tailbone, just above the First Chakra – that is, in the area of the Second Chakra.

So. The Energy <u>resides</u> there – in its "abode" – a "lake" or "well" of Energy waiting to be accessed and utilized. And the Chakra name is thus, to my mind, once again very specific and very apt.

A Related Practice: The Belly "Clench & Slam"

Inhale. Exhale two-thirds of the air out. Pump your belly for a bit; then quickly switch your maneuver: clench your torso and slam that pumped midsection air down the torso into your lower back. Slam it down from the midsection, over and over, down into your tailbone area. Over and over, like a pile driver.

When you have to breathe in again, stop.

See what happens.

This is a yet another method to attempt to "awaken" the pool (or ocean) of "Kundalini" Energy that Yogic theory says resides in the area near the tip of the tailbone.

15

Asvini Mudra

The Truth Behind It

We now go to bottom of torso, again to help Awaken the Energy that lies dormant in front of the tailbone. Asvini Mudra is a primary technique for this. And for taking that Energy UP. And it also acts to clear/calm/open/purify/make better the area at the bottom of the torso, which we might wish to call the First Chakra Area.

The Basics of Asvini Mudra

Asvini Mudra ("ash-vee-nee moo-drah"), is relatively simple. After you have taken a big Inhale, and established a Chin Lock, you hold your breath, and while doing so you clench and release your anal sphincter. Over and over and over, for as long as you can while holding your breath.

Clench and release. Clench and release. You can do it quickly or relatively slowly. You can do it with a deep clench or a shallow one.

You may find it works very well to do your clenchings in groups of threes or groups of tens rather than continuously.

You may do more than one round. More than one round is more potent.

Sending Energy Up

Asvini Mudra is in itself a very effective way to zap Energy up the body.

And, to be more specific, I strongly suggest that you use Asvini Mudra to send Energy up to the <u>back of the head</u>, to what is called the Bindu Chakra at the back of the skull.

Just as Agni Sara (and Nauli) seem to me to have a connection to the Third Eye Chakra, at the front of the skull, Asvini Mudra seems to have a connection to the Bindu Chakra at the back.

Earlier in my Pranayama practice, when I would get into rhythmic clenching in Asvini Mudra, I would quite often feel the Bindu Chakra area throbbing in synch with the clenching. And when I realized this I started, successfully, taking Energy up the back to the Bindu Chakra during Asvini Mudra.

The Bindu Chakra is therefore, in my opinion, from my experience, the appropriate terminus for the Energy sent up. Unless of course you find it possible to take it even higher, to the Seventh Chakra at the top of the skull.

In any event, as you perform Asvini Mudra see if you can feel it go zinging up what seems to be the spine.

Releasing Your Chin Lock

When I perform Asvini Mudra while still holding a Chin Lock, I can often feel Energy tapping up against the Chin Lock. And if I release the Lock even slightly I can then often feel the tapping up in the skull. Indeed, I am even often taken involuntarily out of my Chin Lock when I perform Asvini Mudra. I assume this is so that the Energy can go up into my head and not get blocked at the neck by my Chin Lock. So perhaps try doing it with or without a Chin Lock.

Post-Asvini Mudra

Try if you wish to float your consciousness up into the crown of your head, (your Seventh Chakra). You may want to lift your closed eyes up to enhance this.

Advanced Asvini Mudra: Slow and Deep

To do Asvini Mudra in a more advanced/potent manner try to take your clenchings more deeply up into the anus. Do not just clench the anal aperture, but try to bring the clench up, say, four fingers widths into the anus. When you do your clenching that <u>deep</u> into the anus, and in a <u>slow</u> rhythm, it can seem to be more potent at bringing Energy up the spine.

"Deep Asvini Mudra" such as this is best done slowly. But Asvini Mudra itself can be done very quickly. I currently am able to regularly do 60 clenches per held-breath round, or, occasionally, 100 or more if I go fast. (60, or 100, is the maximum recommended by the experienced Yoga Teacher Baba Hari Dass.)

However, I suggest that you first learn to do Asvini Mudra slowly, as this helps in accomplishing the goal of sending Energy up the spine. (Yet again, the goal is <u>not</u> mindlessly going for numbers. Tom.)

Localizing the Clenching

When you clench your anal sphincter there is usually an accompanying involuntary clenching of the urethral sphincter further forward in the pubic area. You want to try to minimize or eliminate this. There are two physical techniques for doing this that are somewhat difficult for me to explain.
One involves a lifting in the back of the spine just above the anus, so that the clenching is felt more in the rear of the lower torso, which serves to help minimize any sympathetic actions in the urethra. The other, which can be learned, is to clench the <u>rear</u> of the anus.

If you get more adept you can also try to localize in another way by squeezing the right and left sides of the anal aperture, going back and forth.

A final way to learn to restrict the clenching to the anus is to practice going back and forth between squeezing the anal sphincter and the urethral sphincter. It helps make the difference clear and teaches the muscles what to do in each mode. (Thanks to Chris P. for this tip.)

Involuntary Clenching Higher in the Body

When you do Asvini Mudra it will sometimes cause an involuntary clenching of Chakra Areas above the anus.

Thus I myself will sometimes experience a very tight clenching in the Second Chakra Area in the lower abdomen. The area will become hard like a clay pot. And this is often followed by sister-clenchings, consecutively, in the Third Chakra Area at the solar plexus, the Fourth Chakra Area at the heart, the Fifth Chakra Area at the lower throat and the Sixth Chakra Area ("Third Eye Area").

One result of this – if indeed the upper Chakra Areas are affected – is that the shoulder blades may be pulled, involuntarily and quite strongly, down the back.

All these involuntary reactions feel great. At the same time that the affected Areas clench they also seem to calm and open and become unblocked. It even feels like – what are the words I'm looking for – they are becoming energized, are widening, blossoming, becoming empowered.

I posit that perhaps these Energy-Rising activities are related to feelings/inner actions that you will try to make occur voluntarily, which will be discussed In Volume II when the Yoga-Locks, Chakra-Rising and Silent-Mantra breathing techniques are examined.

Why Asvini Mudra on a Held Inhale?

Because it doesn't seem to work after an Exhale.

Asvini Mudra and Root Lock

Some Yogic schools of thought believe that Root Lock, "Mula Bandha," is merely the clenching of the anal sphincter like this, rather than some more complex activity. Asvini Mudra is – to this way of thinking – a more "active" version of Root Lock.

Whatever the case may be, Asvini Mudra can help build a muscular power that may help enable you to take and hold Root Lock. And, on a purely physical level, it is a good practice in that it exercises muscles that often cause problems in old age.

"Asva" means "horse." This technique is named after a similar, more obvious, clenching and releasing habit of horses. Never mind.

Results of Energy-Awakening Pranayama

After completing Agni Sara, and/or Asvini Mudra just sit there and breathe normally. Notice what if anything is going on. See what develops. See if anything kicks in about four or five breaths after you finish.

If phenomena do come, go with them. You may – here or at other points in your session – get an internal levitation, when your feet and sitz-bones and body feel like they are rising up into the air. I believe this is a sign of progress. The learned Baba Hari Dass agrees. So let yourself float. See what happens next.

Again: I believe these practices are designed to help awaken the (Kundalini) Energy that Yoga sources say is stored near the coccyx, so that that Energy can rise up the body, ultimately up to the Third Eye or the top of the head or Beyond.

Asvini Mudra is well-placed at the end of your sequence thus far, because it may in and of itself start a flow of Energy up from the base of the spine – which flowing can then be continued in the Energy-Rising Pranayama which can immediately follow.

And if it has induced such a rising up, great! Notice what happens to the body if the Energy does go up. And notice also where your blocks are.

The "Four Purifications"
Nadi Shodana, Kapalabhati, Agni Sara & Asvini Mudra

I came, through my own personal practice, to the basic Pranayama sequence set forth thus far here – without any knowledge of a similar classical Yogic "purifying" sequence that consists of the four practices listed in the above header, in that order.

So. This Guidebook's sequence to this point has an essential similarity to what may be an ancient Yogic practice. There is most certainly a startling synchronicity.

In this "Four Purifications" practice one starts with Nadi Shodana, then goes on to Kapalabhati, Agni Sara and Asvini Mudra.

Regarding starting with Nadi Shodana, recall that I do advise more advanced practitioners to do Single-Nostril Nadi Shodana, (discussed in Volume II) before doing Kapalabhati. That points at a further synergy with the Four Purifications sequence.

The Four Purifications, (as taught currently by Yoga Teacher Baba Hari Dass), are designed to purify the "Airs" or "Energies," (the "Vayus"), in your upper torso, head, belly and lower torso, as a lead-in to more Pranayama and then Meditation – just as the steps in this Guidebook are a lead into Meditation in your Sitting.

The sequence in which the Purifications are practiced is such that they flow naturally one into the other. As do, I feel, the Pranayama of this Guidebook .

16

Ujjayi Breathing

The Basic Truths Behind It

Ujjayi Breathing is a very important Yogic Breathing technique. It is very, very good, in itself, at bringing Energy up.

From the practice of the previously-discussed Pranayama in your session your Energy channels have been opened and cleansed, and, hopefully, the field of latent Energy in your lower body roused. And so now, with Energy-Rising work like Ujjayi, you take Energy up – or up and down – the channels, (or you enable it to do so). Which purifies you even more.

With Energy-Rising Pranayama you are ridding yourself of blockages, so that you can Flow in synch with the Universe. The practice enables you to achieve an even better Flow in your life.

If you are uncertain what I mean by a life that flows, practice Pranayama consistently for an extended period of time and it will become clear.

And in the immediate future, (that is, in your practice session), Ujjayi will enable your Meditation to become deeper.

Ujjayi can also lead you naturally into other Energy-Rising Pranayama that will be discussed in Volume II.

And finally, note that one of things you are trying to do with these types of Pranayama, is – in Yogic terms – to unite your lower body Energies with your upper body Energies, creating superb integrating abilities. In some Yogic terminologies it is said that you are bringing "Kundalini" Energy up from the bottom of your torso to your head. Or, stated in a more poetic way, you are uniting your lower "Shakti" with your upper "Shiva." Self with Self.

The Basics

With Ujjayi ("Ooh [as in 'ooh-lah-lah']-jai-eee") breathing you close your throat down halfway, so that when you Inhale you make a hissing sound and when you Exhale you make a second (different) hissing sound. Note that there are two distinct, different hissing noises, as you breathe in and as you breathe out.

These sounds have been compared to waves on the seashore or to tree leaves rustling in the breeze, etc. But the description that resonates with many of my students is to call this "Darth Vader Breathing." You simply breathe "heavy," like Darth Vader did in the Star War movies.

You should also feel the Inhaled breath against the back of your upper throat.

As an Energy-Rising Pranayama your Ujjayi Inhale goes <u>up</u> your spine from your <u>tailbone</u> to your <u>Third Eye Area</u>. And then your Ujjayi Exhale goes back <u>down</u> your spine to your tailbone. Over and over. Slowly.

Ujjayi is most easily done with your chin slightly tilted down.

You might consider trying to make the breathing slow and graceful and wavelike.

Ujjayi & Energy Sensitivity

Ujjayi techniques can zoom the Breath and its Energy cousin/ companion up and down your body. Ujjayi Breathing is a very good tool for bringing you to an awareness that Energy is not the same as the breath, but can "ride" it, or be pulled along by it, or be induced by it, or activated by it. Or precede it.

Ujjayi Breathing also gives you intimations of Central Channel Breathing, ("Sushumna Breathing"), a deeper, more subtle experience, where the Breath becomes fined down so much that what you sense feels more like it is just Energy itself – not the breath at all – that is flowing up and down a central corridor. Seemingly, sometimes, all by itself.

Ujjayi and the Spine

Though I say you are breathing up and down the spine, Yogic theory indicates that the channel you are using is an infinitely miniscule ("subtle" rather than physical) channel in the spinal area, the "Sushumna."

I feel, though, that it works better to keep your thinking about this breathing focused on something more concrete and overtly physical, something with which you are more familiar, like the spine itself.

Further, in this version of Ujjayi it may help you in keeping your torso in the proper posture if you visualize the breathing happening <u>just in front</u> of your spine, or, with more refinement, in the front <u>part</u> of your spine.

This is because Ujjayi Breathing does not work well at all if you are hunched over and the spine is rounded. If you are slouched forward the Ujjayi Breath is very much impeded. And the flip side of this is that as you Inhale up with Ujjayi Breathing the spine should become more erect and lengthen, of itself, and the chest and body should open…like a cobra rising.

Ujjayi and Chin Lock

On your Inhale you may wish to take the breath up the spine to the throat, and then, continuing your Inhale, take the breath <u>diagonally</u> forward and up, to the Third Eye Area.

If you are in a Chin Lock this change of Energy direction can be difficult to accomplish. It is to some extent blocked. So, while your chin itself can remain slightly tilted down, you might wish to unlock any Chin Lock you may have unconsciously established, when your Inhale reaches the area of the throat and you wish to take it higher.

Sambhavi Mudra

As you Inhale up the spine to the Third Eye Area a simple but important practice called Sambhavi Mudra can help you a lot. Your closed eyes look _up_ and back _into_ your skull, and you cross your eyes slightly in order to focus them on the space between the eyebrows. At the same time, you may very gently take your eyebrows towards each other, (furrowing your brow as if you were puzzled or squinting, but with a more subtle action).

You may then take your inner gaze further into your head.

Ujjayi Breathing, or some other Energy-Rising work, can by itself lead you into the spontaneous establishment of Sambhavi Mudra.

Yoga Teacher Yogani calls our attention to the fact that establishing Root Lock, ("Mula Bandha"), also can in itself help create Sambhavi Mudra. If you have established Mula Bandha, try to feel the Energy being pushed up the body by the Root Lock all the way to the Third Eye Area. See if the push takes the eyes with it, into the crossed, up-and-in position.

The flip side of _this_ is that establishing Sambhavi Mudra tugs Energy up the spine. You can develop the sensitivity to feel this tugging, a tugging all the way up from the tailbone area. You are, after all, dealing with a connected Energy system.

Stretching the Breath

Recall from the discussion in the beginning of this Guidebook that the word "Pranayama" can be thought of in two different ways.

As "Prana" and "Yama" it can refer to regulation, to restraint of the breath; to harnessing Universal Energy by regulating your breath.

As "Pran" and "Ayama" it can be said to refer to "stretching" or "expansion," (the opposite of "restraint.") And may allude to the expansion of Energy, or the stretching of Energy, as in up from the bottom of the torso to the top of the body.

Ujjayi Breathing is a Pranayama in which you might more easily experience the physical "stretching" of the breath than in others. As you do an Ujjayi Inhale - especially if you have done several prior rounds – the breath can feel like it is being stretched tight and taut as it comes up the torso. And this is an effect you wish to have, as, I posit, the more taut things become the more you are travelling in the direction of moving Energy rather than just Breath. And as you fine things down more and more, you get more and more of that beneficial effect.

Two Notes about Ujjayi Breathing

The root "ud" means "upward" and the term "jaya" connotes "victory." Ujjayi can be translated as "Upward Conquering" Breath or "Upward Victorious" Breath. And indeed, as such, Ujjayi Breathing is a primary technique for bringing Energy up from the lower part of the body to the head.

Ujjayi Breathing is often recommended as the way to breathe during Asana, and can also be very helpful in that context. Yoga Teacher Erich Schiffmann, in his wonderful book, Yoga, The Spirit and Practice of Moving into Stillness, has included a very good discussion of the reasons for utilizing it.

Energy Going Up
Kundalini?

To reiterate: when you hear the word "Kundalini" it is often used in the context of an Energy residing at the base of the spine, in a hugely important storehouse, (an "ocean" or "well" of Energy), in the neighborhood of the coccyx. It can also refer to using Yoga techniques to induce this "Kundalini energy" to rise up.

Kundalini can mean "the coiled one," and it is often represented as a snake. The Energy lies, latent (and therefore "coiled") at the base of the spine. Then, as you do Kundalini-rising work, bringing it up, your body may tend to spontaneously clench, harden, lift and widen, all by itself.

Like a cobra raising up its head and readying itself to strike.

Hence, I posit, the name.

What – Exactly - is Kundalini?

Kundalini is sometimes thought of as a special kind of Energy. Yoga Teacher T.K.V. Desikachar, on the other hand, posits, as did his Father, Krishnamacharya, that there is no separate Kundalini Energy, but that the term refers to the blockages of which you rid yourself in order to be able to utilize Universal Energy more properly. Their interpretation is, I believe: a coiled cobra represents danger, but once it has lengthened out, (risen up), it loses its dangerous coiled stature.

What I myself currently believe is that there is just one Vital/Universal Energy, (or, if you like, "Prana"). No "special" Energies, no different "species" of Energy. But that, for some reason, Energy may tend to be more concentrated in us, and accessible to us from, the area of the coccyx. And we may call that concentration Kundalini.

Sidetrack:
Insight

> With the development of "insight" that comes from steady, concerted long-term practice of Pranayama, you may become able to experience the "Kundalini" well-source of Infinite Energy down in the lower abdomen.

Energy: Upward Flowing versus Compression & Expansion

Desikachar indicates that Energy "flows continuously from somewhere inside us…" and "streams out from the center through the whole body." The Heart of Yoga, page 54. Diagrams of the body, adjacent to his text, seem to site the "center" in the area of the solar plexus.

I am aware that Energy can flow from the "center" and that we can also compress Energy into and expand it from that area – (See the "Gems of the Universe" – Manipura Kriya Pranayama in Volume II) – but the basic flow of Energy, in my experience, and that to which most Guidebooks appear to refer to, begins low.

I believe that Desikachar is also of the belief, as was Krishnamacharya, that Prana is an Energy contained within the body, which can be dissipated out of it, but not brought into it by breathing. As A.G. Mohan, Desikachar's long-time fellow-student under Krishnamacharya's tutelage, indicates: "We cannot acquire more prana from the outside – by breathing it into our bodies, for instance." Yoga for Body, Breath, and Mind, page 159.

Okay. So. We are dealing with Theory, and also with Practices and Results. We may not know whether a certain Theory is right or wrong, but we can know from our Experience which Practices bring what Results – and perhaps we may be content for the time-being with that.

And so, therefore, whatever the case may be, "Kundalini-Rising" or "Prana-Rising" or what I prefer to call "Energy-Rising" techniques, like Ujjayi, are potent.

Side-Note:
Yoga Symbolism

> In regard to the usage of the cobra as a symbol, I find it find it interesting, and perhaps instructive, that both the Lotus, as a symbol of Yoga, (portraying our opening), and the Cobra, (as a symbol of "Kundalini Rising"),

can be used to illustrate the bodily field in which we are working.

Recall that the Seventh Chakra is called the Sahasrara, or Thousand-Petalled Lotus – signifying the blossoming we hope to achieve. Thus the crown of the head can be portrayed to be a blossomed lotus flower on top of a long stem, (our spine), just like a lotus on its long stem. And the Cobra also, rising up and flaring its hood, creates the same schematic; its long stem is its body.

Isn't human imagination and creativity wondrous?

Structure versus Variety

I discuss in this Guidebook the concepts of

> Energy-Awakening Pranayama
> and
> Energy-Rising Pranayama

and in the next volume will discuss

> Energy-Expanding Pranayama

…in an attempt to give some cohesive structure to assist you in your comprehension of a convoluted field. However, as should become more and more apparent, there is much overlap, and infinite variety. Everything being interrelated, how could it not be so.

Note also that there are endless ways to move Energy around your body in order to purify and balance yourself. You may, for example, use Pranayama methods as a starting point or points, and then later in a session explore "Energy Work," (discussed in Volume II), on its own. I urge you to experiment, as soon as your inward sensitivity enables it. This may take time. Be patient.

How to Finish

The Basic Truths Behind "Sitting"

Sitting enables a further knitting together of your Energy system. Healing, Opening, Curing and other benefits may occur as you sit.

Sitting may also take you to places which you need to go to – places to which you were not previously aware you needed to go, but which, when you go there, the need becomes obvious to you.

Sitting for some time just after the active Pranayama portion of a session is thus <u>important</u>. Unless you sit there for a while after doing the active Pranayama you may not feel all the effects of the practice.

These effects sometimes take time to kick in. I consider five minutes of sitting essential – less than that does not give those things that want to happen time to do so. More than that is fine. I currently usually do around 16 minutes, but often only because that allows me to do a potent amount of Bija Mantra work, (discussed in Volume II), or other more advanced practices to be discussed in Volume III.

And perhaps – if you Just Sit and Wait, (Waiting Patiently... <u>Patiently</u>) – you might even perhaps achieve absolute, perfect balance and harmony, and be able to Live There for a while. Ah.

The Basic Truths Behind Lying Down

I strongly believe it is also vital to have a lying-down Perfection/Recovery/Curative Period if you have had a Pranayama session of any considerable length.

You may feel spacey, irritable, weird, discombobulated or excessively floaty, (or all of the above), if you forego Sitting/Perfecting and immediately stand up and go about your ordinary business right after your active Pranayama. You can't go from running 100 m.p.h. to an instant Full Stop. You have to ease into it.

(If you do feel spacey, one thing that you might do is drink some water to ground yourself before you go out into the world.)

If, on the other hand, you lie down quietly for a little while, you will feel light and refreshed when you get up afterwards. Apparently we need to recover from the intensity of the practice, then get our bearings back.

I note that Yogani also insists on the need for Resting/Perfection period. As does B.K.S. Iyengar: "Do not walk or talk immediately after pranayama, but relax in savasana for a time before attending to other activities." <u>Light on Pranayama</u>, page 62.

Also, and very importantly: this Perfecting step can take you even deeper. If you remain lying down quietly for a good while, good things can happen. You can continue, or set in motion, the enhancing/repairing/curing/healing processes.

Why not go straight from Pranayama to lying down, without sitting for a while first?

I don't really know. This just evolved for me. I would get so deep after doing Pranayama that just sitting there and "meditating" seemed the only reasonable follow-on. And I feel that meditating is best done seated.

And then, after Sitting, I would often feel so emotionally wiped out/blanked, so "Wow, what was that!?" that my body demanded some time lying down to recover. And when I did so I discovered that further Purifications occurred.

I do posit however that, because of the importance of Energy flow up and down an erect spine, Sitting for a time before Lying Down/Perfecting is useful to further the Perfecting process. However, I really just don't know. And I am leery of trying to invent reasonings after-the-fact to try to rationally justify things that intuitively seem absolutely correct.

17
Sitting: Meditation Variations

Sitting: Structured or Unstructured

I choose to call this phase "Sitting" rather than "Meditation" or "Sitting and Meditating" simply because I don't want you to feel under any pressure whatsoever to do anything except <u>sit there</u>.

And also because just sitting there is enough to enable further Purification. Your Pranayama has prepared you to receive.

On the other hand, I will set out for your consideration some potent "active" options you can do while you are sitting.

With these options you can be active inside yourself, working Energy with various methods other than Pranayama, methods that are designed to bring you into further purification and/or bliss, and in my experience have been proven to do so.

One final basic thought: Sitting, however done, can ideally feel like a really good Savasana, (Corpse Pose), in that you feel like you don't ever want to come out of it.

Just Sit, Anytime

It bears repeating that you do not have to wait until the "planned end" of your session in order to Just Sit. If you feel like doing so after any Pranayama, do so. There is absolutely no downside to this. Don't fall into the trap of having a previously-formed "must-do" list of Pranayama in your mind, which you feel you must get through during your session. That is a sure way to close yourself off from "happenings" for which you might possibly have more need.

Trust yourself to take you where you need to go.

Sitting and "Meditating"

"Open" Meditation

Because Pranayama prepares you to receive, you can Just Sit and see what happens. See if things come to you of their own accord. I call this being open or "Open" Meditation. You can let the mind wander. Let it rip. Or you can, by your stillness, try to keep it at least somewhat tamped down. You are just there, open to anything.

Seeded or Unseeded Meditation

Alternatively you can (1) try to focus the mind on something. Or, (2) without using a focus, try to achieve a completely blank mind.

This type of Meditation – different from "Open" Meditation – can therefore be "seeded" or "unseeded."

Seeded Meditation involves choosing a focus, something verbal, visual or whatever. Focusing on this "seed" helps drown out the "monkey chatter" of the mind, stilling it. At this point in your session, you should be able to utilize "Om" or more complex Mantras for this purpose if you wish to.

Unseeded Meditation is much more difficult. It involves trying for a complete stilling, without focusing on anything. You can attempt it at this point in your sequence – perhaps after a period of seeded Meditation as a lead-in – because after having gone through several Pranayama your mind may be well tamped-down and ready for it.

Internal Chanting

One "seeded meditation" option you might wish to try is internal chanting. To the best of my knowledge chanting, (both external and internal), has been used by religious groups of all persuasions throughout history, as an effective method to experience spiritual progress.

You might use anything that your religious or cultural upbringing suggests to you. Or experiment further.

I'll mention a personal experience in this area, because I found it so extraordinary. One session, as I was sitting there blank-minded after my active Pranayama, I found myself – to my complete and utter astonishment – internally chanting the famous Indian Mantra called the Gayatri Mantra.

I was astonished because – although I had at one point memorized the Maha Mritunjaya Mantra out of respect for a fellow practitioner – I had not done so with the Gayatri Mantra; I was merely passably familiar with the words from having listened to the exquisite chanting of them by Deva Premal in a multitude of Yoga classes. (And I was aware of their meanings.)

And yet here I was spewing it out to myself, perfectly. And the chanting was effectively taking me up the ladder of deeper meditation.

I am not a Hindu, nor do I ascribe to its tenets. In my opinion, however, one very generic transliteration of the underlying meaning of the Gayatri Mantra might be "Aid us in our Spiritual Practices" – an aim which I should think would be acceptable to most all persuasions.

Why did it arise, in me, at that time?... I have speculated.

For what it's worth, I currently also do internal chanting outside the context of a Pranayama session, as part of my personal Yogic regimen. I do what is called "Japa" – the silent repetition of a personal Mantra. I do the commonly-practiced 108 repetitions, counting them out on a "Mala" of 108 sandalwood beads strung out on a circular string.

Why do I do this? Sources I credit suggest it. It re-dedicates me. And mostly: I have come to find it otherwise <u>empowering</u>.

In any event it must have something going for it; many of the organized religions of the world utilize some form of "prayer beads" and repetition.

I will discuss Japa in a later volume.

Preview

>I also do out-loud chanting in my Bija Mantra work, discussed in Volume II. I do this in both solo and in group practices, loudly or whispering, and have found it extremely effective, in all contexts.

Phenomena

As you sit, all sorts of phenomena may occur. You may feel a pulsing; may see things or feel weird things. Or the body may do things, (like head bobbing), involuntarily. You may experience to some degree – either intensely or just getting an inkling – "internal levitation," where your feet and buttocks feel like they are rising up off the floor and chair and your whole body feels like it is rising up, light as a feather.

Or other phenomena.

Third Eye Area Activation

You may get an interior throbbing or pulsing in the Third Eye Area. This may also translate itself into actual head movement. (You may also of course experience this during Pranayama.)

Activation of the Third Eye Area is said by some to be related to obtaining true wisdom…. (I wouldn't know.)

More "Active" Sitting

Involuntary Asana, "Kriya"

Pranayama can operate, in my experience, to open up your <u>muscular</u> and <u>Energetic</u> blocks, to open frozen and crimped portions of your body to both near-term and long-term healing.

In their book <u>Jivamukti Yoga</u>, Yoga Teachers Sharon Gannon and David Lee have entitled a chapter that deals with Prana and Pranayama "Freeing the Life Force." Just so!

Thus, as you sit, you may be taken to various areas of the body and experience them becoming more unblocked. You may go <u>involuntarily</u> into various little, mini, chair-sitting Semi-Asanas. I call this activity "Kriya." Parts of the body may clench, twist, fold, expand, etc. The Chakras may reveal themselves to you. The <u>face</u> and the <u>breath</u> may go <u>wild</u>. You may experience what I call a "Yogasm." (You'll know it if you get one.) (Oh okay: a Chakra area clenches, clenches, clenches, and then bursts.)

No need to worry about any of this. You are being taken where you need to go. The body knows what it needs. We don't like <u>feeling</u> pain, grief, etc. So we box it in and it becomes entrapped in our bodies. It is basic psychology that emotions get frozen in the body. We want to release them.

They can be released in other ways, of course. For example in massage, when the body-worker hits unknown, (or very familiar), areas of holding. But this works well, too. Pranayama and Sitting are wonderful tools for bringing release. So let things happen. Let your body contort or clench or whatever. These are good signs.

Even if you burst into tears. With all these kinds of things you are releasing deeply-held negativity from the body. You are removing

Blocks. You are breaking through armor and becoming psychologically – and hopefully metaphysically – open and supple.

It is more than worth it to go through the emotional torment of releasing the frozen emotions from your body. Yoga is not necessarily a honeymoon. It can be hell. The Bliss is underneath the Poison. You will emerge, better.

Held Asana/Deep Stretching

You can if you wish consciously assume and hold a body position that will encourage release. I think of this technique as a "Yin" type of Yogic posturing, passive and relaxed, rather than a "Yang" type of vigorous stretching.

The method is simple:

1. While Sitting, slowly let the body sink into a position of your choice.
2. Lock yourself into that position, externally. I think of this as "Bandha," as a binding of myself.
3. Let your breath and mind focus on the area inside the body that is being addressed/worked. Breathe into the area. Slowly and deeply. Put your mind into the area so that you can monitor and encourage relaxation and release.
4. Try if you wish to illuminate the Chakra associated with that area of the body.
5. Stay there for a period of minutes rather than seconds.
6. Slowly – very slowly – come out of the position. This slowness is necessary because the body will have gradually sunk into a very deep stretch.

Two examples of areas of tension and/or soreness that may benefit from this practice are your lower back and your neck/shoulder area.

External Om-ing

External (out-loud) Om-ing can take you deeper in Meditation; it can very nicely enhance your "sitting-there" experience. On the other

SITTING: MEDITATION VARIATIONS

hand, there is some risk of losing your concentration, because you are introducing external sound into your stillness.

If you have any doubt about the purifying abilities of sound, have a Yoga Teacher strike a (well-made!) singing bowl while you are in Savasana or in Meditation. Feel how the sound travels wondrously about, inside the Energy Channels of your body.

Or take a Reiki session in which an experienced practitioner utilizes such a bowl.

(Again, the efficacy of out-loud sound repetition will be discussed in some detail in later volumes.)

There may well be myriads of other word – or sound – repetitions that might equally enhance your Meditation. Om-ing has flowed for me from my Yoga background; it's simply one specific method that I know works for me.

The letters A-U-M represent the audible "Om" sound. And "Om" itself can be said to represent the inaudible (that is, it is heard inside you, not by your ears) "unstruck sound" ("anahata nada") which will be discussed in the Perfection chapter.

There are an incredible number of interpretations of what the three letters of AUM are all about. But like most things that have become set into dogma, accretion after accretion can veil some inner truth that started the whole thing off. Dogma often has flowed, originally, from a solid, specific, commonly-shared, enhancing experience.

So. One way you might use external Oming is to divide your external Om into its component A, U and M parts. After an Inhale, exhale and chant, starting low:

- An "ah" begins and is felt resonating in the lower torso.
- An "owe" – or an "ooo" as in "ooo, that hurt!" – occurs and is felt resonating in the upper torso.
- An "mmm" occurs and is felt resonating inside the head.

There is no AUM sound on your Inhale. It is the silence that completes the picture.

SECRETS OF SUCCESSFUL PRANAYAMA

Notice how well this AUM construct works; how neatly the three sounds fit in with Yogic Up-Breathing from the Coccyx to the Throat and on to the Third Eye Area.

Hint: try chanting the three-part Om while in a headstand, or similarly inverted. Feel it.

Inner Self-Healing Option

Moving on to another alternative: if a part of your body is in dis-ease or in need of repair you can consciously send Energy to that part of the body. And use your mind and breath and Energy to actively heal the area. Or, if you are a bit skeptical, you can just "visualize" the healing occurring.

You might not even have to do this consciously. Meditation might take you places.

These two paragraphs are short ones, but important ones. The Sitting phase promotes Self-Healing.

Further, with time, perhaps try to develop the ability to envision, (or develop in-vision), and visualize the inside stuff of your body – your organs, muscles, bones, etc. – and with your insight help make them harmonious.

A "Christmas Tree" Option

After whatever your last Pranayama was, or during Meditation, light up your Chakras, from top to bottom, or bottom to top. Think of it as if you are lighting a Christmas Tree. Turn on Your Lights. Zing Energy from them, like mini-supernova explosions. Let each Chakra contribute. Let their Energy fill your body. Become a Ball of Purity. Purge areas of Dis-Ease.

Feel fabulous.

A "Dessert" Option

At the end of either your Pranayama or your Sitting, when you think are done…

Inhale a thin, needle-like stream of air up through the roof of your mouth, diagonally up to the top rear of your head.

Then Exhale it if you wish from there into the entire head. Or Exhale it slowly to the Third Eye Area, but don't let the Exhale go out through the Third Eye.

Wow! Do it again!

You may wish then to sit some more.

You can do this at other times, during your Pranayama session or when you are out in the world. Caveat: when out in the world don't let it make you spacey.

Find Your Own Side Trips/Options

Just as in Pranayama, there are myriads of little side trips like these, that you can go on as you Sit. And it's nice to follow along, to new things.

Coming Out of Sitting

Come out any way you want.

One method that might be helpful is to rub your hands vigorously together and then "wash your face" with them, especially the area of your eyes, pressing the heels of your hands against your closed eyes.

This rubbing/washing seems to encourage the eyes to open without undue harshness.

Or: rub your palms and wash, and then cover your eyes with them, taking care to create a full darkness. Then sit there with the heels of your hands covering your eyes, and – perhaps – enjoy.

I currently believe that the beauty of what you may see – as opposed to stark darkness – is an indication of a deeper session.

<u>Neither Here nor There</u>. You can also try, if you wish, what I call "Neither Here nor There." I call it that because that is exactly what it feels like.

You can first turn your hands around so the palms are face down and resting on your thighs. (This seems to help close things down, to ground you.) Or rest your hands in any configuration on your lap.

Next, lower your head down. Open your eyes a bit and focus your vision on the on the black line that is the lower edge of the black area (the back of your eyelids) that fills the top your field of vision.

Do not focus on the blackened area itself: that area – above the dividing line – that is darkened by your eyelids. If you do your eyes will tend to close.

Now, keeping your focus on the dividing line, slowly raise your head. Sit there, working to keep your focus on the dividing line. You are now neither in the room nor out of it.

If your eyes do close at this point, lower your head, re-open your eyes slightly and re-focus, and then raise your head again. You may have to do this a few times.

Be in this mode for as long as you like. I think this is a really nice halfway house – you are in-between being inside yourself and being back in the outside world again. Almost like a third place.

Then lower your head and open your eyes a bit more, and lift your head very slowly again, and sit there.

You can go up and down a few times, raising your eyelid line by degrees, and finally perhaps sitting there with completely open eyes, but completely focusing on the black line – not being there in the room.

Then lower your head one last time, and open your eyes, fully now, and be in the room. Come up in the mode.

I suggest this, or some such technique, as a gentle way to come out of the depths.

And now finally:

NOTICE
how calm, relaxed, light and confident
you are as you sit there

LEARN
to take it with you

Walk Lightly through Life
with a Balanced Flow

18

Lying Down: "Perfection"

The Basic Truth Behind It

This "lying down and doing nothing" phase is <u>not</u> a tacked-on afterthought. It <u>Perfects</u> the work you have just done. It is <u>important</u>.

Again, I strongly believe it is vital to have a Perfection/ Recovery/ Curative type Period if you have had a Pranayama session of any considerable length.

Going Deeper in Perfection

Also, and very importantly: this Perfecting step can take you even deeper. If you remain lying down quietly for a good while, good things can happen. You can continue, or set in motion, the enhancing/repairing/curing/healing processes.

Note that you are not exhausted, nor resting, nor dozing. You are quiet, and – hopefully – you will gradually, or even suddenly, feel <u>different</u>.

You may experience waves of well-being or even bliss wash over you. You lie there, blissfully. An utterly peaceful state has descended on you – physically, mentally and emotionally. You are in a state of complete harmony with life:

Perfecting Connects You…Deeper

The Basics

After completing your Pranayama/Meditation, you lie down (I suggest on your left hand side) for <u>at least five minutes</u>. I strongly suggest ten minutes. Fifteen minutes would be much better. I myself, before I start my practice, pre-set a "Perfecting Phase" timer for seventeen minutes.

Feel free to stay longer, of course – as long as your body wants. Unless you find yourself consistently falling asleep with longer stays.

Note that this lying down is not Savasana, the Corpse Pose that is done at the end of an Asana session. It is related to Savasana, but it is designed to lead to quite different results.

The Mechanics

From Sitting to Lying Down

When your body, or your timer, tells you it's time to come out of your Sitting/Meditation, remember to come out gradually. Immediately looking up, or fully opening your eyes, can be too harsh. It can jolt you "out."

When your eyes are open, slowly get off your chair, or roll over on your couch, and lie down on your <u>left-hand side</u>. (I stand up and walk from my chair to a couch.)

I use a couch because…wait for it…it's much more comfortable than the floor. If you want to use the floor I suggest you might want to put some soft padding down on it.

Why on Your Left-Hand Side?

I don't know. All I know is that only lying on my left hand side works for me after Pranayama; that my body will not let me lie on my right side. It screams at me not to.

So. If lying on the left side seems wrong to you, experiment with your right side or lying on your back. Many of my students don't choose the left hand side. But many do, and…

…the best explanation I can currently discover for why you should lie down on your left side after Pranayama, while, on the other hand, you might want to lie on your right side after Asana/ Savasana, is:

> Lying on the left side opens up the right nostril, the heating/energizing ("sun" or "surya") nostril. And perhaps you want this after Pranayama because you can get so very deep "in" from your Pranayama and Meditation that you have to get somewhat energized again, to get you back to <u>balance</u>.
>
> After Savasana, on the other hand, rolling over and lying on your right side for a while opens up the cooling, calming "lunar," ("moon" or "chandra") nostril. And you want this; you want to continue – and take it with you – the quiet calm of the Savasana, after the "heat" of your Asana practice,

Does this make any sense? Perhaps. I really don't know. But in any event: I am well aware of, and can testify to, the heating and cooling effects of the two nostrils.

In sum: as always, go where <u>your</u> body tells you to go.

Calming Aids

I place several small pillows or cushions at various positions on the couch around my body, (between my knees, behind my low back, hugged to my chest, and under the side of my head).

These are helpful. The cushion against my chest, which presses lightly against the aortic arch, (above the heart), helps to engage my parasympathetic nervous system, which is calming. The pillow under the side of my head – because it presses gently against the carotid sinus on the side of my neck – does the same.

A degree of warmth will also help engage your calming parasympathetic nervous system; as does darkness. You can put a blanket over and/or around your body if you wish. I do.

Darkness for the eyes is of some importance. If you are on your back you can use an eye pillow. If the room itself is not dark, and you are on your side you might fold a headscarf, or some such cloth, a few times so that it forms a band that can be placed around or draped upon the skull, covering your eyes.

Your hands, and especially your feet, must not be cold, (just as in Savasana). For example: I usually do my Pranayama in the early morning in a home heated or cooled to about 65 degrees; but if for some reason it is not that warm, then my hands are too cold and I have more trouble achieving a deep, Perfecting lie-down.

One other thing. I currently posit that what may be the optimal arm position, (arms apart so that the chest is open and receptive), involves having the right arm, (up on top), resting along the side of the body rather than being tucked into the chest-chin area. Or – perhaps less optimal – it can rest out perpendicular to the body. Thus when I lie on my side on the floor, away from my home, I sometimes put a small rectangular Yoga foam block out in front of my chest and rest my right arm on top of that.

Quiet Body, Zinging Mind

Your brain may be very active during this Perfecting Period, not quiet like it may usually be in your lying-down Savasana at the end of an Asana class. That's okay. Immediately after your Pranayama your head needs time to work things out: to process stuff that has been brought up, to get rid of crud.

I feel the work going on is something akin to that involved in psychoanalysis, only with more Expert assistance.

Your body, on the other hand, should feel calm. Notice how limp and quiet and pure it feels, <u>or comes to feel</u>. And this calmness may set in – Boom! – all of a sudden.

Signs of an increased calmness can include an uncurling/release of your palms/fingers, your head becoming heavy like lead weight, or your belly (perhaps even suddenly) losing all anxiety and residing in a heretofore unknown peace.

The calmness may even at some point make you feel all wonderfully sparkly inside, tingly, and/or with an interior lightness – especially in the torso, the chest and the belly, and maybe even the genitals.

Why Five to Fifteen Minutes?

Because the body may not immediately get into that most purely quiet state, as described above.

In my opinion, staying in Perfection <u>at least five minutes</u> is important because the body does not seem to consistently sink into this delightfully light, quiet, calm, deep state of being prior to the five-minute mark. Nor, if other desirable things also happen to you, do they usually do so, or do so completely, in a shorter period of time.

I set my personal timer for 17 minutes for two reasons.

The first is that I have learned that for me it often takes about 10 or even 15 minutes for a calmness/lightness of being to set in, and then to set in more completely. And then one of course wishes to live there a bit. I have, countless times, felt things kick in around the 15-minute mark, and want to give them a chance to do so.

The second is that I noted, time after time over the years, that I started to lose things, consistently, almost like clockwork, at the seventeen-minute mark, and either went into "drifty" land or started thinking about more mundane things. Thus the exactness of my own personal 17-minute timer.

I suggest that you may want to find your own "starting to fall asleep" point and adjust accordingly.

I also suggest using a loud timer/pinger..

"Don't Have Time" for Perfection?

Okay. Next time, make time.

But this time, try Perfecting without lying down, during your Sitting step. As you sit there turn your palms downwards on your thighs. Then just sit there a while like a statue, with your eyes closed or open or half-open.

Again, I consider this a poor alternative. But it is better than nothing. It constitutes a necessary interim between your active Pranayama and getting back into what you may consider "Real Life."

Inducing Torso Calmness

If you have been lying down in Perfection for a good while and you do not feel a delightfully calm, empty effect in your torso, you may want to try to do some work internally to make it happen. How? Try to consciously go more soft, more limp in the lower abdomen. See if that does the trick.

Inducing a More Total Torso Calmness

If you do feel a calm emptiness, even a sparkliness, in a portion of your body, (usually the torso), you may want to try to work internally to make your entire body feel that way. How? Again, try to go even more limp in the lower abdomen.

Or see if you can mentally focus on urging the Feeling to spread to your extremities.

Or. One nice thing about Perfecting is that the Meridians may possibly evidence themselves to you.

Inducing Complete Calm

Let go at all the Chakra points. Do this by consciously visiting each one and allowing it to relax. This induces the entire body to become loose and happy instead of clenchy.

And this translates.

As "scientific" experimentation I have on numerous occasion taken my blood pressure with a portable cuff, both upon lying down into Perfection and after lying there for my 17 minutes. My systolic blood pressure (the higher number) drops as much as 20 points. My diastolic (lower) about 4 points.

Third Eye Visions

After having done years of Pranayama, when the calmness comes to me now during my Perfecting periods, I can then perhaps expect my Third Eye Area to become "visually" active and maybe also expect to have some "vision-type experience."

This happens often enough now that it has come to feel perfectly normal to me. So much so that I sometimes feel – irrationally – <u>deprived</u> should it not happen in any particular session.

(Again, becoming enamored of phenomena is a Trap. Your session was not a "good" one or a "bad" one because of what did or did not occur. Every session is a good one – as long as you Keep Practicing with Persistence.)

As for the details: allow me to just reiterate that at some times there is a tunneling effect with a circle opening up at the end of the tunnel, and with a vision inside that circle. Or – said differently – a grayish, circular surround appears, (often tunnel-like), with a small, cleared circular area in its center, and inside that clear area will be some utterly clear image, either static or moving – and most always, <u>but not always</u>, of something of which I can make no sense at all of. Recall what was said previously in the discussion about the symbolic Sri Yantra.

The presence of a surround should alert you to the fact that what you are about to experience, or are seeing, is a "vision."

Briefly, then, here are just two not-necessarily-representative examples of clear images I have seen:

> A vision of my arm and my hand, in black and white, like a photograph; and – fluttering while resting on the back of my hand – a butterfly, in beautiful color.

> A vision of a shrub, all green, with a small red patch in its shrubbery.

The beauty and clarity and the "It's there and I'm seeing it"-ness of these kind of visions separates them from any other experience I have had in life.

Or: I may experience a perfectly-defined, luminous white dot; or a white dot and a black dot (similar to the Chinese Yin-Yang symbol). You may also experience things like this by staring at a flame for a time, then closing your eyes, (a practice called "Trataka").

Or: more rarely, an eye looking back at me. A human eye. Not a reflection of my own eye. A human eye.

Or, extremely rarely thus far, a full face.

You cannot successfully mandate, or even urge these types of things to happen. But if you let yourself be in a state of "I'm okay either way, if something comes or not," then they may come.

Hearing the "Unstruck Sound"

During Sitting or Perfecting you may hear the "unstruck sound," the term for a sound that you hear not with your ears but deep inside your head, which arises spontaneously there, apparently unbidden, apparently without physical source.

For me thus far it has been comparable to the beeep-beeep-beeep warning signal sound a truck makes when it is backing up, only less strong and with less noticeable intervals – almost as though it's pulsating.

Or like the humming sound of an electrical transformer or electrical lines.

Or like a very faint bell being rung so repeatedly that it's nearly a constant sound.

Or like the sound of a small bee.

(It is not the same sound you get with "ringing in the ears"/ tinnitus)

This internal sound is likely to be overwhelmed by external sounds. Yet another reason to practice in the early morning, in complete quiet.

What is the meaning of hearing this sound?

"Unstruck sound" is the literal translation of the Sanskrit term "Anahata Nada." Other translations might be "sound current" or "audible life-stream." Some Yogic thought thus considers this sound to be the sound of the Energy of the Universe. And considers "Om" ("AUM") to be an audible representation of it.

There is in fact an entire branch of Yoga called "Laya" or "Nada" which deals with attempting to experience inner sights and sounds. You can if you wish, as you are in your Sitting step, try to intensely focus on listening inside.

Experiencing this sound is perhaps, at the least, a sign of a deep Perfecting. If you experience it be sure to notice how things look to you when you come out.

A Relevant Side Trip into Meaning: Fourth Chakra

Note that the Heart Chakra is called "anahata" or the "center of the unstruck sound."

Why?

I suggest that you get "deep" and then "om" silently into your heart.

(The Heart Chakra is also supposedly "activated" by doing a Pranayama which resembles bees humming – "Brahmari" Pranayama – which I do not discuss in this Guidebook.)

Coming Out

When you are finally ready to come out of your Perfecting, try lying there with your eyes open for a minute or two before getting up.

If your eyes don't want to open, stretch out your two sets of index and middle fingers, make them rigid, and then wiggle them vigorously about, like tuning forks, while you curl your ring fingers and little fingers, forcing their fingernails against the underside of your thumb tips. (You make a "Vee" sign.) That should help.

I happened on this particular hand-positioning and its effect myself, but note with some interest that it is close to the positioning of the Indian "Pran Mudra," which is supposed to give you energy, and be good for your eyes.

Try to keep your eyes open but soft. Be aware that this initial opening – the exact moment you let your eyes open – is a "prime time" for "visions."

And as you lie there with your eyes open you may quite possibly notice effects from the Session.

Some Examples:

>Colors may be more <u>Vivid</u>.
>Everything may look <u>Crisp</u>.
>Everything may look like it <u>Fits</u>.
>
>You might see everything as an <u>Interlocking Construction</u>, as an absolute <u>Geometric Perfection</u>.
>You may feel you are <u>Welcome</u>.
>That you are <u>In Place</u>.
>That you <u>Belong</u>.

You may even... <u>Sense Life Where Before You Have Not</u>.

Draw your own conclusions.

Post-Perfection

As you walk around afterwards – if you did get "deep" in that day's session – everything may look beautiful. "Oh! Look at the chair!" "Look at the phone!" "Look at the note pad!!"

And as you stand up and walk around, notice how loose and light and airy you feel. And how calm, confident and empowered. Your body should feel clear, strong and calm. You should feel full of grounded willpower.

Thus established, go about your Work.

These good things, and others – the full "near-term" effects of the Pranayama Session – are in my opinion allowed to come more into fruition during the Perfecting period. They seem to need it in order to fully manifest.

And, the more you go into Pranayama the more you might be able to carry these feelings with you into your day. Rather than having a wondrous session only to have things immediately dissipate afterwards.

So. Nice. Very nice. A wonderful way to go about your life. But these physical and mental feelings are <u>side</u> <u>effects</u>. Not – Not At All – the important thing.

The test of whether your Pranayama practice is effective is <u>not</u> how you feel right after it, or even during your day; it is <u>not</u> how effective you thought things were going while you were doing it; it is <u>not</u> whether you did or did not experience any neat phenomena. It is:

How Your Day Flows
How Your Life Flows

This is what Yoga is for. The Whole Thing.
You are linking yourself up to, yoking yourself to, Power.
You are doing this to better – <u>at the least</u> – <u>your</u> life.

Pranayama is Life-Transforming

Health Benefits of Yoga & Pranayama

Yoga is, in so, so many ways, an "enriching experience." It enables living well. But this Guidebook is not intended to recount all of the numerous, (and well-chronicled), physical, mental, emotional and spiritual benefits claimed for it.

I do however wish to briefly touch on a few points apropos to Pranayama, both by itself and in conjunction with Asana and Meditation.

These are points on which I feel I have enough personal experience to at least opine.

Freedom from Sickness

On the physical level, Yoga is, first and foremost, a system that promotes all-around health.

I've been teaching Yoga for thirteen years now, (five days or more a week during most of that time), and it is <u>extremely</u> rare for me to miss a class due to illness. This despite being in close contact with a number of students each week.

I do bring home little gifts from them: a sore throat here, a sniffle there. In most every case, however, the twinges are gone, magically, the next day. I can count on less than my two hands the times I have been "sick" over all these years. I am in fact surprised and disappointed when I actually do come down with something. (And so – when I do – I lose it.)

One explanation of this protection, on the physical level, is that the invigoration of the Energy systems of the body by Asana and Pranayama includes invigoration of the immune system.

Life Extension & Anti-Aging

This was discussed at the very end of the Nadi Shodana chapter.

The opinion of Tirumalai Krishnamacharya – whom I have ample reason to believe is trustworthy – was that asana practice is "useful for maintaining wellness, but pranayama [is] necessary for maximizing life span." <u>Krishnamacharya, His Life and Teachings</u>, A. G. Mohan, page 57.

Krishnamacharya's life bore witness to his belief. He lived to be 100 years old. He practiced Pranayama daily and credited Pranayama for his longevity. Mohan, who knew him well, believes – I think reasonably – that Krishnamacharya would have lived much longer had he not suffered a hip fracture at age 95. He refused hip replacement surgery, and was therefore greatly limited in his physical activities post-accident. The orthopedic surgeon who examined him at the time and who recommended the hip replacement stated "His heart and lungs are like a man thirty years younger. He may be ninety-five years old, but he is as fit as an active sixty-five-year-old man." Mohan, page 83.

Krishnamacharya, by the way, is considered a seminal source of many of the aspects of what we nowadays consider "Hatha Yoga" to be. His students K. P. Jois, B.K.S. Iyengar, T.K.V. Desikachar (his son), A. G. Mohan, Srivatsa Ramaswami and Indra Devi, and their students, etc., etc.... Etc. – have been factors in the expansion of Yoga outside the Indian subcontinent.

Krishnamacharya considered Pranayama the most important of the "eight limbs" of classical Yoga. I do not feel it accidental that I have been drawn towards its practice and propagation. (And, I am also grateful to C. Brennan for giving me the Mantra for this work: "Worldwide Pranayama.")

Pranayama & Calm in Your Life

The stereotype of a Yogic practitioner is someone who is an unnaturally calm person. I myself, however, tend towards an unfortunate, intense, burning ferocity - Yoga, however, and especially Pranayama, have tempered this to a great extent, sprinkling calmness and happiness more and more over my life, bringing some measures of balance and acceptance.

The physiological reasoning here, perhaps, is that both Asana and Pranayama (1) strengthen the body's nerves and (2) release tensions that we hold in our body, inducing calm.

Yes, I believe that. But I also believe it's much, much more than that. Pranayama somehow brings calmness into the activities of your life. The stressors tend towards fading out of it. You are left with more of the good stuff. More and more and more calmness descends gradually into your life.

Again, bad things do happen. And sometimes Really Bad Things. But you become harder to rattle. And, when you do get really rattled, you are more likely to bounce more quickly back into balance. You trend towards just calmly and quietly fixing things. You accept yourself as a flawed, normal human being, and you acknowledge your inevitable mistakes and work from there.

You calm, whether you want it or not. A calmness, perhaps "unnatural" in the context of your previous life, descends on you, willy-nilly.

One of the most easily felt results of Yoga, and one that is thus much commented upon, is this enhanced serenity.

And. What I have experienced, and what gurus have told us, is that you first, eventually, become a happier person…
      …and then – (<u>they</u> say) – a blissful person…

Weight Control from Pranayama?
The "Lean and Stringy" Yogi

Another common stereotype of a Yogi is that of a lean and stringy person. What's the truth behind this?

One truth is that a lot of the lean and stringy "yogis" you see in Yoga ads were in fact already lean and stringy dancers and gymnasts.

But again, I can relate from my personal experience. (I am not a lean and stringy person, and never have been.) Decades ago, I was for a time a soccer referee. I loved it, and in fact I injured myself from too much refereeing. I blew out the soles of my feet. For years I had plantar fasciitis of varying severity; for a few months I could not even bear to walk on concrete.

Unable to do aerobic exercise, my weight ballooned.

It was only when I took up Pranayama – and only after I took it up very seriously – that I experienced a relatively rapid and relatively effortless weight loss that has brought me, in my middle age, to much less than my college-age belt-size.

Why is this? I think there are three possible, perhaps interrelated, explanations.

The first – advanced in some Yogic literature – is that because Pranayama brings so much Prana (Energy) into you, you can live more on that Energy, needing less food.

The second is that Yoga both calms you and fills you up, so there is less need for emotional eating. I personally do know that the more Pranayama I do the less I feel the stronger urges to eat, and the more I am satisfied with meals of less calories and bulk.

The third explanation is that as Pranayama engenders Flow – that is, as you flow more and more in synch with and as part of the Power of the Universe: (1) your willpower is substantially increased, and (2) barriers to what you want do to are, quite naturally, lowered – both of these because what you want to do is what you should be doing.

I currently subscribe, with perhaps a bit more certainty, to this third explanation. We all know what we need to do to lose weight. Pranayama empowers us to do it.

In any event, my testimony, as of today is: deep and persistent Pranayama <u>enables</u> beneficial weight loss.

And – sigh – the "unfortunate truth" flip side of this is that belly fat will keep you from <u>full</u> achievement in both Asana and Pranayama. There should be no sugar-coating of this important fact. I know this from personal experience. And the school of Yogic thinking – which I respect – based on the teachings of Krishnamacharya, concurs:

> [T]he teacher will need to observe if the student has the necessary prerequisites for a pranayama practice – good posture, a straight spine, and a taut abdomen.
> Yoga Teacher A. G. Mohan
> <u>Yoga for Body, Breath, and Mind</u>, p 164

Respiratory Capacity

If you practice Pranayama for a period of years, your respiratory capacity will become much greater. Period. The muscles that you use in breathing strengthen tremendously. This has to be good.

In my Yoga classes I teach a variation of a pose called "Lion." We all stand, hunching forward slightly, putting our hands on our bent, widespread knees. Then – taking our tongues out and down, and looking up with and crossing our eyes – we take a huge Inhale and then roar like lions, as loud and as long as we possibly can.

It's a tremendous stress-buster and invigorator. I usually teach it when my students are starting to drag from overly-strenuous Asana work. (Try it when you are stressed-out inside your car some time.)

But here's my point. I was never, for years and years, anywhere near being among the longest-roaring lions. But then one day during my ninth year of teaching I discovered, to my utter surprise, that I had outlasted everybody.

This appealed, unfortunately, to the "extreme Pitta" in me. I had the class do it a second time – and this time my "best-lung-ed" student decided, Oh, Okay, she'd put her heart into it this time.

Nevertheless, my capacity had, quite obviously, grown. I believe that Kapalabhati, and also the torso-clenching aspects involved in some Pranayama, were among the most potent of the Pranayama practices involved in bringing about this growth.

Pranayama, Asana & Energy

Asana & Pranayama Recap

Asana and Pranayama are Brother and Sister. They work together to open your Inner Body. They operate Hand in Hand. Pranayama unlocks Asana for you. It shows you the way.

Over the years, Asana have become to me – as Yoga Teachers and other commentators have mentioned – more and more Outer Manifestations of an Inner Opening. An Exterior Freedom that reflects an Inner Freedom, an Inner Space.

Asana unblocks your armored and tight areas, and helps allow your Chakras to blossom. A well-composed Asana opens you up inside. In a really good Asana you may feel like you are being turned inside-out. Likewise, sometimes, in a good Pranayama.

I am convinced that Pranayama has opened me much more to Asana. I believe Yoga Teacher B.K.S. Iyengar has been quoted as saying something to the effect that Pranayama acts like a jackhammer on tight muscles. My experience is in fact such.

If you practice both Asana and Pranayama your body can become light and airy inside – a wonderful way to feel. My guess is that this is due at least as much to the removal of psychic blockages and crimpings within you, to the lessening of your psychic burdens, as to the physical twistings, bendings and stretchings you have done.

Pranayama only after Proficiency in Asana?

In order to fully experience Pranayama do you have to be prepared for it by having had a previous Asana practice? Even: many years of it?

My students' reactions to the Pranayama portions of my classes, workshops and private lessons vary greatly:

<u>Some Students</u> get it, almost fully, almost instantly. Most of these seem to be experienced in Asana or, if not, in Meditation.

<u>Most Students</u> get at least a "Wow!" factor – they experience some sort of pleasant, new-found-land, altered state. "I feel like I just joined a cult!"

<u>Some Students</u>, however, just don't get there. They're all at sea. "What's it *for*, Tom?" "I guess I'm just not good at *breathing*."

With time though, if they persevere, my experience has been that things do begin to dawn on these students. Um, nearly all. Sigh.

I believe one main theory as to why an Asana practice may be considered a necessary preparation for Pranayama, (a theory strictly adhered to by some contemporary schools of Yogic thought), is that the Nadis, (the Yogic term for the body's internal Subtle Energy Channels), must be first, over time, preliminarily purified and prepared by Asana in order for the Pranayama to work to full effect.

I myself had ample Asana before I got into Pranayama to any significant degree, so I cannot speak to this from personal experience. I currently believe, however, that the correct interpretation of Yogic history is that the first Asana were purely seated poses, designed <u>solely</u> to enable lengthy sitting for meditative practices. (Asana is derived from the Sanskrit "as" which refers to "seat.")

In any event: it is essential to have a <u>strong</u>, <u>open</u> body in order to sit for an extended period of time without your body's needs intruding on your Pranayama and/or Meditation. And an Asana practice will help give you this strength and openness. So prior Asana is – in fact – very helpful.

Pranayama During Asana?

Some Yoga schools advise, or mandate, Ujjayi Breathing during Asana. Or advise/mandate some sort of ratio-ed, controlled breathing. And all schools of which I am aware emphasize breathing through the nose. I think all these things serve good purpose. Anything is better than huffing and puffing like steam engine, clenching everything.

I have experimented with Ujjayi in Asana and like it a lot. Besides its internal effects, it is settling. The hissing noise is something to focus on, providing a sort of contemplation. And, if you start to strive too much, physically, in a pose, the change in the sound of your hissing breath can serve as a more vivid wake-up call than your normal breath.

That said, I am not wedded to Ujjayi in Asana. And that I am not could just be my particular Yogic background.

I do also enjoy and benefit from, utilizing Mantra in Asana.

And I do feel strong benefits when I utilize Yoga Locks during asana.

And finally, I am also fond of the conscious bringing of Energy up from the Kundalini area to the center of the torso during Asana, which I think can be a potent addition to most poses. It is both energizing and steadying.

Pranayama: Before or After Asana?

Pranayama After Asana

My experience has been that Pranayama may be practiced just as effectively after a session of Asana as it can as an unrelated, stand-alone practice. Or even more effectively.

I believe there are at least two reasons for this. First, an Asana session will lessen the amount of tension you are holding in your body. And second, Asana, because it is physical exercise, opens up your respiratory system for easier breathing.

I myself can very successfully practice Pranayama just 10 or 15 minutes after an hour-long Asana practice.

That said, going immediately from vigorous Asana (such as backbends) into Pranayama doesn't work. You are way too jazzed up. Better instead to end your Asana practice with some quieting poses, (forward bends or some sort of shoulderstand-plough-fish-front bend sequence), and/or lie down for a bit in Savasana, before Pranayama.

I have however found that it is extremely difficult for the students in my classes, once they are lying down in Savasana, to get up out of their cozy, wonderful relaxation and start doing Pranayama – and I have for the most part given up trying to browbeat them into doing it.

So instead, in most of my classes: immediately after Asana, (well, okay, there is a hiatus while everyone in the class gets blankets, puts on socks, constructs their sitting position, etc., etc., ad infinitum), I give everyone some basic Pranayama.

And then, after Pranayama, those who wish to can take Savasana. The rest continue with some more Pranayama and with their Sitting and Perfecting periods, which can, in part or in full, take the place of Savasana for them. In my advanced classes many more students opt to remain seated. They've gotten it.

Pranayama Before Asana

I can quite happily do an Asana session starting just twenty or thirty minutes after the end of a Pranayama practice of more than an hour, with no problems. Moreover, my Asana seem to me to flow especially nicely after Pranayama; the body seems set up for Asana by Pranayama.

That said, I don't teach this way in class. Most of the studios and students I have encountered are, at this point in time, primarily interested in Asana: "Woo-hoo! Let's get to it! Let's do the workout!!"

Sigh.

Working with Energy

I am convinced that in both Asana and Pranayama we are working with our interior portions of Energy, with interior Energy Lines and Counter Energy Lines. That we are working for the Union of Opposites, and for the resultant <u>Balance</u>, for the perfect Balance of the <u>Flows</u> from which we receive <u>Harmony</u>:

Balance
Harmony
Flow

As we become more and more balanced and harmonious, and can flow, it is not too much to expect, I believe, for us to become better and better iterations of ourselves; to slough off our constricting skins, and emerge, more.

In that regard – at the very beginning of this work I mentioned Wisdom, Power and Compassion. I think it is best to strive for Compassion – and let the Universe take care of Power and Wisdom.

Other Pranayama Books?

I have read ancient and modern sources. I do not discount modern sources and rely solely on quote-unquote "scriptures" of ancient lineage. To me it stands to reason – there now being billions of people on our Earth – that, statistically, some of us have, at the least, just as good a chance as the ancients of getting things right.

I hesitate to single out individual Works or Teachers for fear of leaving out equally credible sources of which/whom I am not as yet aware. That said, those Teachers whose works I have mentioned favorably in this book are those, I feel, worthy of your consideration.

But okay: I won't completely duck a valid question. If you as a beginner have the inclination to delve deeper: the collection of lessons by Yogani, Advanced Yoga Practices, a good part of which deals with Pranayama, and Richard Rosen's two books on Pranayama, all mentioned earlier, are where I would at this point be inclined to send you.

Approaches to Pranayama will always be different. But so very, very many of these two Teachers' words and teachings mirror or echo my own experience. As they should: the essence will, of course, always be the same.

True Confession: I myself read and re-read one book over and over, because I tend to get so wrapped up in newly discovered Pranayama techniques that I forget how nice it is to revisit the basics – and also because I do not want to forget all the nuances…

This Guidebook.

The Big Picture

We exist in an Energy World.
We know of it, from experience.
But we don't have a complete handle on it.
Yet.

Rigidity & Simplicity

Rigidity and Simplicity are the antitheses of Life.

Asana and Pranayama unlock us from rigidity, awaken us to our vast, interlocked Energetic world. Open us like flowers blossoming. To receive.

We yearn, however, for simplicity and certainty. Doubt is not comfortable. We long for interpretations that are nice and neat; that hang together; that connect and comfort all over, like cozy blankets. And then when we find them, we become overly attached to them.

Is this yearning, this longing, this disability, human nature, set? Are we destined to forever repeat the religious-based crimes of the previous eons? Or can we transcend?

Asana, Pranayama and Meditation are magnificent tools to achieve transcendence.

Portals to Experiencing the Energy World

I consider – from my own personal experience – Massage, Acupuncture and other Body/Energy work as allied art-sciences to Pranayama and Yoga.

Example One. One day Maria, a substitute masseuse at a facility, gave me an incredible massage. I of course wanted to book her again, but was unable to make contact. Weeks later, standing in a parking lot outside a Safeway grocery store, I felt, for the first time ever, Energy surging up from the earth into my body. I was astounded.

I walked into the Safeway in a daze. Maria was inside, shopping there also. We re-connected. I had many, many sessions with her after that. She wasn't just a masseuse or a body worker, but an Energy-Worker, and her work took me to places inside me that I never imagined existed, it opened me to inner worlds of incredible beauty.

Example Two. My first experience with acupuncture was when I tried it to try to relieve pain in my <u>right</u> leg. The practitioner began sticking needles into my <u>left</u> leg. As she did so, I felt Energy begin to flow up the left leg, cross the pelvis, and flow down into my right leg, balancing me.

I told her what I was feeling. She explained, with some surprise, that Yes, That was the idea. As with Pranayama, she was working with Energy in the body.

Regarding the Energy channels in the body: for a long time I could not understand how the Yogis of India could have come up with what I feel is their ludicrous assertion of the existence of "72,000" or "320,000" or whatever "Nadis," while the Chinese, plainly at least equally astute, could come up with just a handful of equivalent "Meridians." Then I learned that the Meridians most discussed are just the main avenues; that Chinese Energy-thought has "sub-Meridians" that encompass the entire body, like the Nadis do.

Ah. Connection.

So – in a like manner to Yoga – acupuncture and different types of massage by experienced Energy Workers have opened me to new worlds of the Energy, within my body and otherwise.

At some point in the future I would hope that this whole, now-somewhat-disjointed panoply is tied together in an accepted, interrelated Energy schema.

Georg Feuerstein, our foremost contemporary Yogic scholar, agrees:

> While Western science is still struggling to find explanations for such phenomena as acupuncture meridians, Kundalini awakenings, and Kirlian photography, yogins continue to explore and enjoy the pyrotechnics of the subtle body, as they have done for hundreds of generations. ....
>
> I believe it is only a matter of time before the emergent scientific paradigm will generate a comprehensive model of bioenergetic fields that can also help us understand and vindicate some of the stranger practices of Hatha-Yoga.
>
> <u>The Yoga Tradition</u>, p 351

How sweetly apt is Feuerstein's word, "pyrotechnics."

As of now, however, I think we are like the blind men groping at the different parts of the elephant and coming up with differing descriptions of its essence.

One other – (half-formed, but when has that ever…) – thought. I believe current scientific thought is in some sort of agreement that the known Matter in the Universe is in reality only about 10% of all the Matter in the Universe, and that the other 90% is "Dark Matter," of which we know little to nothing about but are able to deduce its presence.

Perhaps the idea that discoveries will tie together our currently incomplete consensus regarding the nature and charts of our "interior" Energy – and its linkage to "exterior" Energy – may not be utterly far-fetched, nor those discoveries far distant. Like the transition of our knowledge from flat-earth to round-earth, discovery may well perhaps burst, unexpected, upon us.

Your Work

As mentioned before, this is not in any way a comprehensive encyclopedia of Pranayama. There is an infinite variety of it for you yourself to discover.

Further, progressing in Pranayama is a fascinating, never-ending Exploration. I learn more each and every week. I do my practice with a pen and pad at my side. I look forward to the new things that will come to me. I feel like a small sponge upon whom a fire hose has been trained.

So. I am therefore curious about, and very much look forward to seeing, what a revised version of this book might look like years down the road – how similar or dissimilar it may be to this particular snapshot in time.

In any event, and wherever you yourself are eventually led, know that what has been offered to you here, as a starter, WORKS. My individual experience, and the feedback of my students, over years, are both testimony that the individual Pranayama and the Sequences that are set forth here are indeed wonderfully potent, and that these things happening to us, both while in and because of Pranayama, are Experienced Truth.

But...
    This Guidebook just gets you into the Neighborhood.

**Your Work
is to Find the Home
where You should Be**

I hope your path evolves with grace.

Namaste.

This Work is dedicated to
Y. Fedotova and T. Krishnamacharya

> Even, as I breathe,
> Comes an angel to their keep.
> Surely, if this is,
> Promises are mine to give you...
> Mine to give...
> –Enya, "Angeles"

Namaste. Namaha.

Our Aim:

"What are people for?"

K. Vonnegut

Printed in Great Britain
by Amazon